Tweets, Likes, *and* Liabilities

Online and Electronic Risk to the Healthcare Professional

BY MICHAEL J. SACOPULOS AND SUSAN GAY

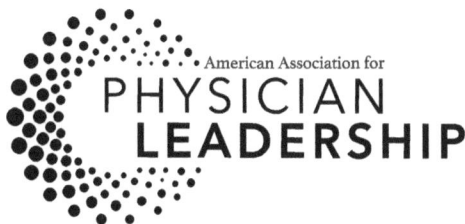

American Association for
PHYSICIAN
LEADERSHIP

Published by **American Association for Physician Leadership, Inc.**
PO Box 96503 | BMB 97493 | Washington, DC 20090-6503

Website: www.physicianleaders.org

AAPL books are available at special quantity discounts to use as premiums and sales promotions, or for use in corporate training programs. For more information, please write to Special Sales at journal@physicianleaders.org

This publication is designed to provide general information and is sold with the understanding that neither the author nor the publisher is engaged in rendering legal, accounting, ethical, or clinical advice. If legal or other expert advice is required, the services of a competent professional person should be sought.

13   8 7 6 5 4 3 2 1

Copyedited, typeset, indexed, and printed in the United States of America

PUBLISHER
Nancy Collins

EDITORIAL ASSISTANT
Jennifer Weiss

DESIGN & LAYOUT
Carter Publishing Studio

COPYEDITOR
Pat George

TABLE OF CONTENTS

ABOUT THE AUTHORS

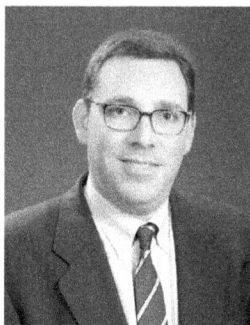

MICHAEL J. SACOPULOS, JD is the CEO of Medical Risk Institute (MRI), a firm that provides proactive counsel to the healthcare community to identify where liability risks originate and reduce or remove these risks. Mike's unlawyerlike pragmatism and clever wit make him a sought-after speaker by national specialty societies such as MGMA national and state chapters, and trade associations.

Mike is General Counsel for Medical Justice Services where he is tasked with keeping the organization's members out of meritless lawsuits. In a fit of madness, Mike agreed to work with a Lloyd's of London firm, to write the first cyber insurance product designed exclusively for healthcare industry. He has written for *Wall Street Journal*, *Forbes*, *Bloomberg* and many publications for the medical profession. In 2016 he was selected as the 2016 "Lawyer of the Year" in the practice area of Medical Malpractice Law for Indiana by "Best Lawyers." Michael also won the 2012 Edward B. Stevens Article of the Year Award for MGMA. Mike is the co-host, along with Cheryl Toth, of the podcast, www.soundpracticepodcast.com.

Mike attended Harvard College, London School of Economics, and Indiana University/Purdue University School of Law. A maniacal birder, Mike has travelled to several of God's forbidden places in search of species to add to his "Life List." Reach him at msacopulos@medriskinstitute.com, or www.medriskinstitute.com.

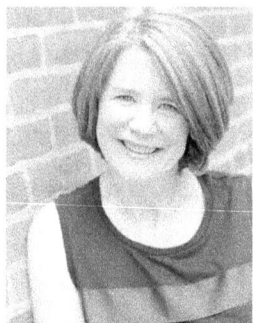

SUSAN GAY is a medical publisher and content strategist. Known for her foresight and vision in creating ground-breaking publications, she has published several hundred books, journals and multi-media products over the past 30 years. Many are still market leaders today. Her creative imprint can be seen in such pioneering works as the 5-Minute Clinical Consult and the Netter Collection reference works. She also served as president of the American Medical Publishers Association.

As the digital era began to fundamentally reinvent medicine and health care delivery, Susan created her own firm to focus on multi-channel content creation, and helping publishers and societies extend their existing portfolios. She has worked with many companies and societies including: American Medical Association, American Academy of Pediatrics, MediMedia, LWW, Elsevier, and Thomson-PDR.

In 2012, Susan switched from publisher to author, first partnering with Kevin Pho, MD (www.kevinmd.com) as co-author of *Establishing, Managing, and Protecting Your Online Reputation*, published by Greenbranch Publishing. Her role in this book is a natural follow-up, given the greater significance that social media plays in healthcare today.

Susan graduated from Presbyterian College (SC) and received a Master's degree from Emory University. She and her husband live in Bryn Mawr, PA. She can be contacted at: susan.infobrand@comcast.net.

ACKNOWLEDGMENTS

This book is the product of many kind individuals. As children we all learned not to judge a book by its cover. This is good advice when looking at our names on this cover. Many other people's efforts have gone into generating this book. You hold a product of Greenbranch Publishing in your hands. The editors, designers, and staff at Greenbranch are exceptional in dedication and quality. We wish to specifically thank our publisher, Nancy Collins. She was always helpful, smart, and encouraging, all while displaying the patience of Job.

Because there are two of us, we each have people who have helped us with this project or influenced our careers.

∿

In many ways this book is an effect long separated from its causes. While writing this book two of my most important friends and teachers died. Susie Dewey was a lifelong friend and my seventh grade English teacher. In ways both patent and latent she is in these pages. Professor Lawrence Jegen tried to teach me tax law. He ended up teaching me many things outside of the tax code. I miss them both on a daily basis.

Cheryl Toth is a tremendous writer, friend, and colleague. Her assistance in creating parts of this book cannot be overstated. Thanks, Tothie. Background research by Matthew McDavitt of the National Legal Research Group was helpful. Finally, many thanks go to Dawna Hoffman who typed and commented upon my drafts. This book was made better by you asking, "What is this really supposed to mean?"

To my wife and children, thank you for your patience and understanding as I wrote. To my brother and law partner, I hope this explains the reduction in my billable hours. To my parents, thank you a lifetime of love, education, and support. **M.S.**

∿

This book came about in part because of another book I co-wrote with Kevin Pho, MD on social media and online reputation management, also published by Greenbranch. I am grateful to Kevin for his guidance through the ever-changing landscape of social media in medical practice. He has been an inspiration to many in this field.

I have spent my entire career in the medical publishing industry and I am thankful to many leaders in the industry who supported my ideas and gave me many opportunities to pursue new and original concepts. I learned a great deal from many people over the years and I'm especially indebted to Ted Hutton, John Gardner, Tom Mackey and the late Sheila Carey. But it's doubtful I would have ever entered this field at all had it not been for the early teachings of one gifted physician, my father, the late Dr. Brit B. Gay, Jr.

Finally, my role in this project would not have been possible without the unwavering support of my husband, Jonathan Andrews. **S.G.**

Dedication

To healthcare providers that take care of patients everyday despite constant harassment from attorneys and third-party payors.

Patients, Physicians, and Social Media: The State of the State

Few would question the importance of social media in the lives of our fellow Americans. Cell phones have robbed Clark Kent of a changing room, and Google is the new Oracle of Delphi. It is in this cyber world that physicians and healthcare executives must find their way. This book serves as a map to this world.

Many healthcare providers view social media as a marketing vehicle to attract patients but also a potential source for HIPAA breaches. While both of these are true, social media offers physicians many more opportunities and risks. This book will enable practice managers to understand the security, privacy, and compliance issues created by technology and social media. We will give practices the knowledge and tools to reduce liabilities and exploit cyber benefits.

A recurrent theme throughout the book is that cyber risks are new and often unexpected and unforeseeable. But this is not a book of worry and paranoia. Cyber celibacy is not a good strategy. Consider this book your guide to medicine in the cyber age.

Monitoring and responding to reviews is an imperative for practices today. The impact of a physician's online reputation extends far beyond just giving patients the opportunity to read reviews. It extends to the credentialing process, will increasingly be connected to satisfaction scores and reimbursement, and can even have unforeseen effects on potential litigation.

Many physicians and practices are reluctant to embrace social media because of concerns about the risks it poses. The advantages of information sharing and interactivity must be weighed against privacy concerns and the creation of a permanent electronic record. From better clinical results to decreased malpractice risks, social media can provide tremendous benefits to practices.

In other words, it shouldn't be ignored!

SOCIAL MEDIA AND THE HIRING PROCESS

Not only is social media increasingly used to recruit and screen employees, but once hired, staff members' personal use of social media may affect the practice. Thus, policies are needed to outline the expectations of employees' social media use outside the practice.

Given that social media platforms such as Facebook, LinkedIn, and Instagram have essentially become diaries or logbooks of the user's daily interactions extending back years, it has become increasing common for employers to delve into the social media pages of employee candidates as a means of uncovering details about the applicant's personal habits, activities, quirks, and personalities. Social media platforms also provide an opportunity to see if a candidate is truthful when preparing his or her resume.

However, such forays into the job candidate's social media accounts do not come without risks. Since 2012, roughly half of the U.S. states have enacted legislation expressly barring employers from directly (or often even indirectly) accessing employees' or job applicants' private social media accounts. At least four additional state legislatures currently have bills under review to extend protections to their citizens. We've included a state-by-state listing of social privacy legislation as well as numerous related case studies in this book.

Beyond these regulations is the fact that these investigations may also trigger various civil rights and antidiscrimination claims. Social media accounts supply employers with a wealth of "protected class" information that may not be utilized legally in an employment context. Details regarding the candidate's inclusion in a legally protected class bring up the specter of discrimination and the hiring process regardless whether the employer in fact utilized the information during the hiring process.

To help you minimize your risk, we've covered "best practices" for the hiring process and provided guidance for establishing sound social media policies for your employees.

SOCIAL MEDIA AND POLICIES IN THE HEALTHCARE PRACTICE

Professional ethics and etiquette form the core of the *Model Guidelines for the Appropriate Use of Social Media and Social Networking in Medical Practice*, put out by the Federation of State Medical Boards. Despite the lengthy official title, the guidelines are brief, straightforward, and succinct. They offer a firm foundation on which to build the specifics of your practice's social media policy. Following them demonstrates your willingness to adhere to "industry standards" for cyber security, online behavior, and patient privacy.

For reference, the *Model Guidelines for the Appropriate Use of Social Media and Social Networking in Medical Practice* appear starting on page 49 of this book. You and your staff would be wise to review them, adopt them as policy, and cover them in your employee training.

The *Model Guidelines* address doctor-patient relationships first, noting that in the digital era, such a relationship may begin online rather than in person. This means that both the doctor and the patient must be able to firmly establish their respective identities when communicating electronically. Of equal importance, physicians must be aware that standards of medical care *do not change* based upon the means of doctor-patient communication.

Physicians must always be aware that even online interactions that appear innocuous or trivial may violate the doctor-patient relationship. Medical professionals should never use their position to develop personal relationships with patients—online or off.

When it comes to discussing medicine online, the *Model Guidelines* are bracingly firm: Never do so on personal social media! Stick to professional online platforms, such as Doximity. This professional platform for physicians allows you to exchange HIPAA- compliant messages and images and discuss the latest treatment guidelines and medical news.

When posting content, you must be aware that it may be widely disseminated and could "live" in the digital world forever. That's a sobering thought, since anything you post is also subject to misunderstanding, misinterpretation, and being taken out of context.

The security, privacy and confidentiality of the material is your responsibility as well.

The *Model Guidelines* also deal with professional behavior. The key takeaway here is to separate your personal online presence and your professional online presence. Keep material on personal sites personal and professional sites professional. Make sure they are always separate and unique. The same goes for email. Use professional email addresses for professional communication and personal email addresses for personal communication. Do not allow the two to overlap—no mixing and matching!

When it comes to HIPAA violations, there are, sadly, plenty of examples available to serve as cautionary tales. Some seem like innocent mistakes that just about anyone could make. Others are so egregious that those involved appear to be willfully inviting the wrath of regulators and malpractice attorneys. We'll provide case studies in this book showing HIPAA violations that offer valuable lessons for anyone dealing with patient privacy issues in the digital age.

YOUR PRACTICE WEBSITE

What could be more legally benign than a basic practice website? A medical practice website is straightforward, noncontroversial, and displays only the facts.

Your website is a marketing asset. But it's also a source of potential liability. The content and links on your website need to comport with your state board of medicine's requirements. HIPAA, copyright, and trademark violations, lack of encryption and security, and failure to make the site accessible for those who have visual or hearing impairments are just a few of areas that physicians often don't think about when they are in the throes of designing a site.

We'll tell you why developing your website on a do-it-yourself platform is not a good idea. In Section III, we show you how to conduct a risk assessment with appropriate web development vendors.

The HIPAA Omnibus Rule requires all business associates, no matter how big or small, to follow the same rules your practice does when it comes to the privacy and security of protected health information (PHI). That means if a web developer does not have a breach policy and procedure, or does not provide initial and annual HIPAA training to its employees and independent contractors who work on your website, or does not use a web host that is HIPAA compliant, technically speaking, your practice is not HIPAA compliant.

If you haven't updated your BAA in recent memory, contact a healthcare attorney to ensure it meets all of the HIPAA Omnibus Rule requirements.

The Federation of State Medical Boards (FSMB) guidelines mentioned earlier impacts web content too. But, individual state boards of medicine also have ethics rules that apply to a practice's website. Many of them are holdovers from the pre-digital age. From example, some states prohibit physicians from using patient testimonials. Other states do not allow the posting of before and after photographs, even with patient consent. Certain states prohibit the use of the generic term, "board certified," requiring that you provide the name of the specific board that has certified you.

Given this patchwork of state boards rules that apply to website content, you should consult your licensing board for specific guidance.

The guidance in this book will help you understand the liability issues associated with your practice website, and give you tools and suggestions to make sure your site doesn't turn into a law suit any time soon.

CYBERSECURITY

Are you certain that all staff members and physicians know how to recognize a phishing email? Is every mobile device, tablet, and laptop encrypted and password protected? Have you prepared your team to recognize and handle a social engineering scheme?

Most offices are short staffed. The appointment schedule is overflowing. Many practices lacks professional management. Thus, the answers may be "no" to at least one of these questions.

Unfortunately, cybercrime has hit a fever pitch these days. The prevalence of electronic health records (EHRs), cloud-based applications, and the Internet of Things (IoT) has increased the vulnerability of healthcare data, with 2017 called the "worst year ever" for cybersecurity incidents, according to the Online Trust Alliances' Cyber Incident & Breach Trends Report.

Preparedness efforts such as developing policies and procedures and implementing ongoing employee training are essential to helping any size practice avoid an attack that compromises your systems and results in stolen data or ransom demands.

In Section III, we detail practical action steps that a hyper-busy physician or practice administrator can take to plug common preparedness gaps and develop the policies, procedures, and training necessary to maintain digital security measures. According to leading cybersecurity expert James Scott, the most common weak spots in healthcare information security aren't due to a dearth of technical security features or tools, but human error.

Preparing the practice and employees to identify, avoid, and take action when they recognize cyber issues such as phishing, social engineering attacks, and ransomware schemes is a vital part of cybersecurity. Business associates should also have appropriate policies and procedures in place to protect your data. Remember, the HIPAA Omnibus Rule holds physicians accountable for ensuring that the business associates they contract with have appropriate privacy, security, and breach protocols in place. We break down the tasks here by focusing on the biggest risks first.

Social media policies are essential from both a security and human resources management perspective. They should be shared with employees upon hire and on an ongoing basis.

A mobile device policy is often missing in physician practices. Given the number of smartphones, tablets, laptops, and other devices used by physicians, other clinicians, and staff, this is another policy that is extremely important. We cover the "best practice" recommendations for mobile devices as well.

Once policies and procedures are complete, the next step toward preparedness is training physicians and staff. Effective security training is different than training for other needs. Unlike other forms of training that are "one and done," cybersecurity training is much more effective when it is delivered in shorter sessions, more frequently, with ongoing reminders to keep employees on alert to phishing, malicious attachments and other scams.

The goal is to imprint in employees' minds that your practice takes cybersecurity very, very seriously—because the threat to your patients' privacy is very, very real.

Employees are a practice's weakest link in the effort to maintain cybersecurity. Reduce the risk by being prepared and maintaining awareness. Develop customized policies and procedures that reflect your practice's specific circumstances. Use the practical techniques from this book to create training material and job aids that go beyond generic HIPAA modules.

ONLINE REVIEWS AND RATINGS

These days, one cannot underestimate the power of online reviews.

Studies have shown that 82% of patients now use online reviews to evaluate physicians, and that 72% of patients use them as the first step in finding a new doctor.

The growing use of online reviews has caused many healthcare providers to consult firms who offer services specifically in online reputation management, and to make it a key part of their marketing budget. Although these firms use software to monitor online reviews, it is difficult to remove a negative review. Instead, best practices today call for healthcare providers to manage and improve their online reputation proactively. It's a great example of how an ounce of prevention is better than a pound of cure.

In recent years, patient satisfaction has gained increasing attention from executives across the healthcare industry and from the federal government, first as part of a hospital's HCAHPS scores starting 10 years ago and shortly thereafter with Medicare basing its reimbursements in part on these measures.

Because of the emphasis being placed on patient satisfaction today, it can no longer simply be relegated to periodic surveys, ignored altogether, or simply monitored by an outside vendor. The growth of the ratings business online has made it easier for patients to describe their healthcare experiences in detail and to express their satisfaction—or lack of satisfaction. Increasingly, the online rating sites are the places where the patients' opinions will be aired.

Why not be proactive and address these issues up front? Soliciting patient feedback, listening to patients talk about both the positive and negative experiences, and using those observations to improve your practice is a good way to safeguard your reputation.

Patient satisfaction is increasingly being seen as a vital metric of performance, similar to measures of access, quality, and costs of care. As such, it can be transformative in the culture of healthcare.

Yes, negative reviews are inevitable, but resist the temptation to ignore this trend because having *no* reputation is as bad as having a negative reputation. Nowadays, when potential patients do a search and find several physicians' profiles that meet their criteria for specialty or geography, do you really want yours to be the one with no information about your practice? A straightforward and positive online presence could boost your business now, as more patients find you and decide to make an appointment with you based on what they've read.

If you want to determine the impact of social media on your practice, you can use a metric every business uses to measure the impact of its investments of time and money: the return on investment (ROI). Simply ask new patients how they found you. You may find that a growing percentage of new patients coming to your office are there because of information they found about you online.

One study showed that a significant percentage of patients are willing to overlook important factors, such as cost or inconvenience, in favor of positive online reviews. Forty-eight percent of patients are now willing to go out of network for a better reviewed doctor!

So, maintaining a positive reputation online through careful management of reviews impacts the bottom line of your practice. The other economic benefit of increasing positive online reviews is that it helps the practice maintain overall high ranking in online search results. When reviews are combined with a strong social media presence, good search engine optimization, and a good website, your practice can quickly rise to the top of the leading search engines like Google, driving traffic back to your website and more patients to your practice.

But, just as there are rules that govern physician behavior online and using social media, there are "best practices" that are unique to healthcare providers in responding to online patient reviews. We'll cover these best practices in upcoming chapters.

CONCLUSION

With the explosion of social media options, and the dependence on digital tools in medical practices, healthcare professionals should have a strong working knowledge of both the opportunities that these tools provide, as well as the risks associated with them. We all live online every day. Opting out is not a solution! This book provides clear, helpful guidance to medical practices engaging in the cyber world.

Social Media and the Ghost of Employees, Present and Future

Van Allen, a headhunter, must have been anticipating a handsome placement fee when he matched a newly minted psychiatrist with the hospital. But things did not go as planned. A quick review of the physician's Facebook page was revealing. There were photos. "Pictures of her taking off her shirt at parties," Allen said. For reasons best left unexplored, her behavior seemed habitual. "Not just on one occasion, but on another occasion, and then another."[1]

Oh my.

As you might imagine, the hospital did not hire this psychiatrist. "Hospitals want doctors with great skills that provide great services to communities," Allen explains. "They don't want patients to say to each other 'Heard about Dr. Jones? You got to see those pictures.'" It is difficult to disagree with Allen on that point.

Given that social media platforms such as Facebook, LinkedIn, and Instagram have essentially become diaries or logbooks of the user's daily interactions extending back years, it has become increasing common for employers to delve into the social media pages of employee candidates as a means of uncovering details about the applicant's personal habits, activities, quirks, and personalities. Social media platforms also provide an opportunity to see if a candidate is truthful when preparing his or her resume.

Plowing through sterile, carefully crafted resumes is only the first step in the costly and time-consuming hiring process. Then comes the candidate's carefully worded answers to the employer's questions. "My biggest weakness? Well, I would have to say that I am a perfectionist. I just want to get everything absolutely perfect for my employer." If the candidate were being honest he would say, "My biggest weakness? Well, I have terrible interpersonal skills and I smoke way too much weed." Since that type of honesty is rarely forthcoming in an initial job interview, employers understandably want to use social media to develop a better understanding of a candidate, knowing that they may see an entirely different person on Facebook or Instagram or Twitter.

However, such forays into the job candidate's social media accounts does not come without risks. Some risks are minor, such as the vague hint of nausea that I experience when I see a candidate's glowing review for Mamma Mia 2. More significant risks come from the fact that since 2012, roughly half of the U.S. states have enacted legislation expressly barring employers from directly (or often even indirectly) accessing employees' or job applicants' private social media accounts. At least four additional state legislatures currently have bills under review to extend protections to their citizens.

But the troubles do not stop there. Aside from the direct liability imposed by states actively barring employers' intrusion into job candidates' and employees' social media accounts, these investigations may also trigger various civil rights and antidiscrimination claims. Social media accounts supply employers with a wealth of "protected class" information that may not be utilized legally in an employment context.

Details regarding the candidate's inclusion in a legally protected class bring up the specter of discrimination and the hiring process regardless whether the employer in fact utilized the information during the hiring process.

EQUAL EMPLOYMENT OPPORTUNITY COMMISSION AND FEDERAL ANTIDISCRIMINATION LAWS

A deep dive into a candidate's social media posting may reveal certain traits that may not, under federal law, be considered in the hiring process without potentially triggering liability. Employers may not discriminate against employees based on the following traits:

- Sex, now expanded to encompass sexual orientation and gender identity (Title VII of the Civil Rights Act of 1978, 42 U.S.C. §§ 2000e *et seq.*);
- Race, religion, color, or national origin (Title VII of the Civil Rights Act of 1978, 42 U.S.C. §§ 2000e *et seq.*);
- Age (40 and over) (The Age Discrimination in Employment Act, 29 U.S.C.A. § 621, *ff.*);
- Disability (physical or mental) (The Americans with Disabilities Act, 3 U.S.C.A. § 421);
- Pregnancy (The Pregnancy Discrimination Act of 1978, 42 U.S.C. §§ 2000e(k), amending the Title VII of the Civil Rights Act of 1978 prohibition on sex discrimination to encompass the pregnant);
- Military service (current military service obligations, such as monthly National Guard duty, or former service-people recalled to active military duty) (Uniform Services Employment and Reemployment Rights Act, 38 U.S.C.A. § 4311); and
- Medical status or genetic health risks (The Genetic Information Nondiscrimination Act, 42 U.S.C.A. § 2000ff-1).

These laws are enforced by the Equal Employment Opportunity Commission or EEOC, a federal agency that administers and enforces civil rights laws addressing workplace discrimination.

The problem with these protected class categories is that, once a hiring officer uncovers such details outside of the normal job candidate evaluation process, even if the employer ignores such protected class information in the hiring process, the mere availability of such details to the employer during the hiring process can prompt a rejected candidate to initiate a claim. "I know the reason they didn't hire me is because my child is disabled." "I know the reason they didn't hire me is because I said in my blog that my depression has kept me from being as productive as others."

Unfortunately, the EEOC may find it difficult to accept that such personal characteristic data did not play a role in the hiring decision.

The EEOC may be right in thinking that internal bias may consciously or subconsciously be colored by a candidate's membership in a protected class. In a 2013 study by Carnegie Mellon University, 4,000 fake resumes were submitted for real job postings and corresponding personal protected class data was made available online concerning the bogus job candidates. It was discovered that applicants who affiliated with the Muslim faith solely on fake online platforms, not in written resumes, were 13% less likely to receive a callback compared to non-Muslim candidates with equivalent credentials and experience. This led the authors to conclude that "online disclosure of certain personal traits can influence the hiring decisions of U.S. firms."

Similarly, a study conducted in Belgium recently sought to determine how even superficial Facebook content might impact hiring decisions. The authors sent identical fictitious applicant resumes linked to fake Facebook profiles to real job openings, with the sole difference being the fake Facebook profile photos showed randomly selected levels of attractive people. The fictitious candidate with the most favorable Facebook profile photos received approximately 21% more positive responses to his/her application in comparison to the candidate with the least favorable profile picture. The authors of this study concluded that the likelihood that it was chance that those with attractive photos were favored for interviews over those with less-attractive photos was about 38%.

Another study from Europe surveying hiring personnel usage of Facebook and LinkedIn as sources of information on job candidates concluded that "profile pictures on Facebook … tend to [be read by hiring personnel for]… signals of extraversion and maturity… creat[ing] the risk that common selection biases occur even before the first interview."[2]

What apparently remains unknown, however, is whether there is a significant difference between traditional, pre-Internet job candidate appearance bias versus similar selection bias based on social media photographs or information. Certainly, with social media platforms like Facebook, the risk of selection bias is almost certainly greater, given that Facebook for most users functions as a virtual diary of their activities, conversations, likes and dislikes, political views, religious and disability status, and the like, allowing curious employers to delve into personal details never before so readily available.

This realization has prompted civil rights advocates such as the American Civil Liberties Union to decry employer intrusion into job candidate social media accounts. The ACLU argues that employers requesting such access is akin to invading the applicant's home or listening into their telephone conversations, and that such access should be legally prohibited.

STATE LAWS ON SOCIAL MEDIA PRIVACY IN THE HIRING CONTEXT

Parallel to the federal antidiscrimination statutes, more than half of U.S. states have codified laws, most enacted between 2012 and 2015, restricting employer access to job applicant social media accounts and, in many cases, explicitly barring employers from requesting such access directly (i.e., by demanding login and passwords) or indirectly (i.e., by requiring the applicant to scroll through their social media accounts with an employer representative watching, a practice colloquially termed "shoulder-surfing," or by forcing applicants or new hires to "friend" an employer representative).

I feel compelled at this point to reveal that the above restrictions do not apply to parents. Those of us with teenagers should feel free to "shoulder surf" and be unapologetically invasive of our teenager's social media accounts.

State statutes vary in their scope, applicability, and penalties/remedies, and thus, it is helpful to review a chart summarizing their content by state. A law firm has produced a very helpful chart that tracks the specific scope and penalties associated with each state's iteration regarding social media privacy[3]; this chart is reproduced in Table 1. In addition, at least four states–Georgia, Hawaii, Massachusetts, and Minnesota–currently have bills before their legislature comprising draft social media privacy laws broadly similar to those of other states.

Additionally, on April 28, 2016, House Bill H.R.5107 — 114th Congress (2015–2016), titled the "Social Networking Online Protection Act" was introduced at the federal level. The description of this proposed federal statute is "To prohibit employers and certain other entities from requiring or requesting that employees and certain other individuals provide a user name, password, or other means for accessing a personal account on any social networking website." This bill has not yet moved past the introduction stage.

This suite of state laws governing employer access to candidate/employee social media accounts are new, and a thorough search of Westlaw reveals that there is no case law yet interpreting them, so guidance on the issue of compliance is necessarily speculative.

A leading case on the dangers of employer usage of social media to vet job candidates is *Gaskell v. Univ. of Kentucky*, No. CIV.A. 09-244-KSF, 2010 WL 4867630 (E.D. Ky. Nov. 23, 2010). In that case, the plaintiff, C. Martin Gaskell, an internationally respected British astronomer, sued the University of Kentucky after not being hired as the director of an astronomical observatory, despite being the lead candidate, according to the University of Kentucky's own admission.

After narrowing the pool of applicants to seven, as part of the selection process, the university hiring committee performed an Internet search of the finalists and the search on Gaskell revealed an article in which Gaskell espoused creationist beliefs. Members of the hiring committee expressed concern that such beliefs were incompatible with a leadership position in science, as creationism was unsound based on the scientific method. Two committee members "admitted that [they] would be 'worried' every time Gaskell, if selected as Observatory Director, would be let out in public" that he would embarrass the university by giving religious opinions incompatible with science and thus injure the reputation of the university. Therefore, a secondary candidate was offered the position of observatory director (*Gaskell*, No. CIV.A. 09-244-KSF, 2010 WL 4867630 at *5).

Gaskell filed a complaint with the EEOC charging the university with religious discrimination and thereafter filed suit. Though the university argued that its decision not to hire Gaskell was based on doubts about Gaskell's ability to strenuously advance the scientific process (and not merely because he was a creationist), after the university lost a motion for summary judgment on the discrimination issue, the university settled with Gaskell and without admitting wrongdoing, agreed to pay Gaskell $125,000.

Another case on the pitfalls of social media use by employers is *Nieman v. Grange Mut. Ins. Co.*, No. 11-3404, 2013 WL 1332198 (C.D. Ill. Apr. 2, 2013). In *Nieman*, an insurer, Grange, had begun a search for a candidate to fill an open vice president position at their company. Nieman was interviewed by phone by Grange hiring personnel, and Grange claimed that it eliminated Nieman for the position during that phone consultation, alleging that Niemen was long-winded and overly colloquial about the job duties. Nieman argued at trial that Grange disqualified him discriminatorily after it accessed his LinkedIn profile and, from his college graduation date, determined that he was over 40 years old.

At trial, the court found that prior to Nieman's interview, a previous candidate—a man who was over a decade older than Nieman–had been offered the position but had declined it. In the end, the court granted the defendant employer's motion for summary judgment on the discrimination issue, stating that the plaintiff's case was based entirely upon speculation.

Thus, the *Nieman* case is a cautionary tale that even a disgruntled job candidate's factually baseless claims of "protected class" discrimination can drag unwitting employers into costly legal battles upon the mere accusation of improper usage of social media data in the making of hiring decisions.

The collection of state laws largely barring employer access to job candidate/employee social media accounts reportedly were spurred in reaction to a legal dispute in Maryland. In November 2010, Robert Collins reapplied for his job as a corrections supply officer with the Maryland Department of Public Safety and Correctional Services (MDPSCS) after a leave of absence taken earlier that year. According to MDPSCS policy, before employees could be rehired, "corrections officers who have had a break in service [must] undergo a recertification, . . . [which] includes fingerprinting, a renewed background check, and [an] interview." (Letter from Deborah A. Jeon, Legal Dir., ACLU of Md., to Sec'y Gary D. Maynard, Md. Dep't of Pub. Safety & Corr. Servs. 1-2 (Jan. 25, 2011)).

During his recertification interview, Collins was asked whether he used social media, and when he replied that he used Facebook, he was asked for his Facebook username and password. *Id.* at 2. Collins was told that job candidates were required to provide social media login information as "a standard part of the [Department of Corrections'] process for hiring and recertification ... to enable the [Department] to review wall postings, email communications, photographs, and friend lists, in order to ensure that those employed as corrections officers are not engaged in illegal activity or affiliated with any gangs." *Id.*

The ACLU complained about the practice and the agency subsequently amended its policy to ask candidates to instead log in during interviews, a tactic later deemed problematic in the various state laws addressing this privacy concern (as merely and indirect method to obtain access to the same information).[4]

STATE-BY-STATE CHART

State	Are personal social media accounts covered by the law?	Is personal social media defined?	Is there a private civil right of action?	Are current employees covered by the law?	Are attorneys fees available?	Does the law cover colleges and universities?	Are public employees covered by the law?	Exceptions for investigations of employee misconduct?
Arkansas	Yes	Yes	Not Mentioned	Yes	Not Mentioned	Yes	Yes	Yes
California	Yes	No	Not Mentioned	Yes	Not Mentioned	Yes	Not Mentioned	Yes
Colorado	Yes	No	Yes	Yes	Not Mentioned	Not Mentioned	Yes Law Enforcement Agencies Exception	Not Mentioned
Connecticut	Yes	Yes	Yes	Yes	Yes	Not Mentioned	Yes Law Enforcement Agencies Exception	Yes
Delaware	Yes	Yes	Not Mentioned	Yes	Not Mentioned	Yes	Yes	Yes
District of Columbia	Yes	Yes	Not Mentioned	Not Applicable	Not Mentioned	Yes	Not Applicable	Not Applicable
Illinois	Yes	Yes	Yes	Yes	Yes	Not Mentioned	Not Mentioned	Yes
Louisiana	Yes	Yes	Not Mentioned	Yes	No	Yes	Yes	Yes
Maine	Yes	No	Not Mentioned	Yes	Not Mentioned	Not Mentioned	Not Metntioned	Yes
Maryland	Yes	Yes	Yes	Yes	Not Mentioned	Not Mentioned	Yes	Yes
Michigan	Yes	Yes	Yes	Yes	Yes	Yes	Yes	Yes
Montana	Yes	Yes	Yes	Yes	Not Mentioned	Not Mentioned	Not Mentioned	Yes
Nebraska	Yes	Yes	Yes	Yes	Yes	Not Mentioned	Yes Law Enforcement Agencies Ecception	Yes
Nevada	Yes	No	Not Mentioned	Yes	Not Mentioned	Not Mentioned	Not Mentioned	Not Mentioned
New Hampshire	Yes	Yes	Not Mentioned	Yes	Not Mentioned	Not Mentioned	Not Mentioned	Yes
New Jersey	Yes	Yes	Yes	Yes	Yes	Yes	Yes Law Enforcement Agencies Exception	Yes
New Mexico	Yes	No	Not Mentioned	No	Not Mentioned	Yes	Law Enforcement Agencies are Not, Does Not Mention Other Public Employers	Does Not Apply

State	Are personal social media accounts covered by the law?	Is personal social media defined?	Is there a private civil right of action?	Are current employees covered by the law?	Are attorneys fees available?	Does the law cover colleges and universities?	Are public employees covered by the law?	Exceptions for investigations of employee misconduct?
Oklahoma	Yes	Yes	Yes	Yes	Not Mentioned	Not Mentioned	Not Mentioned	Yes
Oregon	Yes	Yes	Yes	Yes	Yes	Yes	Not Mentioned	Yes
Rhode Island	Yes	Yes	Yes	Yes	Yes	Yes	Yes	Yes
Tennessee	Yes	Yes	Yes	Yes	Yes	Not Mentioned	Yes Law Enforcement Agencies Exceptions	Yes
Utah	Yes	Yes	Yes	Yes	Not Mentioned	Yes	Yes Law Enforcement Agencies Exceptions	Yes
Vermont	Yes	Yes	Not Mentioned	Yes	Not Mentioned	Not Mentioned	Yes Law Enforcement Agencies Exceptions	Yes
Virginia	Yes	Yes	Not Mentioned	Yes	Not Mentioned	Yes	Yes	Yes
Washington	Yes	Yes	Yes	Yes	Yes	Not Mentioned	Yes	Yes
West Virginia	Yes	Yes	Not Mentioned	Yes	Not Mentioned	Not Mentioned	Not Mentioned	Yes
Wisconsin	Yes	Yes	No	Yes	No	Yes	Yes	Yes

State	Is shoulder surfing prohibited?	Must admin. requirements be exhausted before filing suit?	Exceptions for information available on the public domain?	Are employer issued/ business related accounts covered under legislation?	Are employers prohibited from retaliating?	Is there an exception to comply with regulations?	Is there an exeption to implement policies on use?	Is there an exception to discipline for tranfer of confidential info?	Is there an exception to monitor?
Arkansas	Unclear	Not Mentioned	Yes	No	Yes	Yes	Not Mentioned	Not Mentioned	Yes
California	Yes	Not Mentioned	Yes	No	Yes	Yes	Not Mentioned	Not Mentioned	Not Mentioned
Colorado	Unclear	No	Yes	No	Yes	Yes	Yes	Yes	Not Mentioned
Connecticut	Yes	Unclear	Yes	No	Yes	Yes	Yes	Yes	Yes
Delaware	Yes	Not Mentioned	Yes	No	Yes	Yes	Not Mentioned	Not Mentioned	Yes
District of Columbia	Yes	Not Mentioned	Yes	Not Applicable	Yes	Not Mentioned	Not Mentioned	Not Mentioned	Yes
Illinois	Yes	Not Mentioned	Yes	No	Yes	Yes	Yes	Yes	Yes

State	Is shoulder surfing prohibited?	Must admin. requirements be exhausted before filing suit?	Exceptions for information available on the public domain?	Are employer issued/ business related accounts covered under legislation?	Are employers prohibited from retaliating?	Is there an exception to comply with regulations?	Is there an exeption to implement policies on use?	Is there an exception to discipline for tranfer of confidential info?	Is there an exception to monitor?
Louisiana	Not Mentioned	Not Mentioned	Yes	No	Yes	Yes	Yes	Yes	Yes
Maine	Yes	Not Mentioned	Yes	No	Yes	Yes	Not Mentioned	Not Mentioned	Yes
Maryland	Not Mentioned	Not Mentioned	Yes	No	Yes	Yes	Yes	Yes	Not Mentioned
Michigan	Yes	Yes	Yes	No	Yes	Yes	Yes	Yes	Yes
Montana	Yes	Not Mentioned	Yes	No	Yes	Yes	Yes	Yes	Not Mentioned
Nebraska	Yes	Not Mentioned	Yes	No	Yes	Yes	Yes	Yes	Yes
Nevada	Not Mentioned		Yes	No	Yes	Yes	Not Mentioned	Not Mentioned	Not Mentioned
New Hampshire	Not Mentioned	Not Mentioned	Yes	No	Yes	Yes	Yes	Yes	Yes
New Jersey	Not Mentioned	Not Mentioned	Yes	No	Yes	Yes	Yes	Yes	Not Mentioned
New Mexico	Not Mentioned	Not Mentioned	Yes	Not Applicable	Not Mentioned	Not Mentioned	Yes	Not Mentioned	Yes
Oklahoma	Yes	Not Mentioned	Yes	No	Yes	Yes	Not Mentioned	Yes	Yes
Oregon	Yes	Not Mentioned	Yes	No	Yes	Yes	Not Mentioned	Not Mentioned	Yes
Rhode Island	Yes	Not Mentioned	Yes	No	Yes	Yes	Not Mentioned	Not Mentioned	Yes
Tennessee	Yes	Not Mentioned	Yes	No	Yes	Yes	Not Mentioned	Yes	Yes
Utah	Not Mentioned	Not Mentioned	Yes	No	Yes	Yes	Yes	Yes	Yes
Vermont	Yes	Not Mentioned	Yes	No	Yes	Yes	Not Mentioned	Yes	Yes
Virginia	Not Mentioned	Not Mentioned	Yes	No	Yes	Yes	Yes	Not Mentioned	Yes
Washington	Yes	Not Mentioned	Not Mentioned	No	Yes	Yes	Yes	Yes	Yes
West Virginia	Yes	Not Mentioned	Yes	No	Not Mentioned	Yes	Not Mentioned	Yes	Yes
Wisconsin	Yes	Yes	Yes	No	Yes	Yes	Not Mentioned	Yes	Yes

BEST-PRACTICE ADVICE FOR USING SOCIAL WHEN HIRING

Employer use of online information in making hiring decisions is a potential minefield, as hiring personnel may consciously or unconsciously utilize facts gleaned from these sources to screen out candidates based on state and federally protected class traits. The EEOC itself supplies some advice on the topic, even if such information is not "official" guidance (emphasis added):

"Renee Jackson of Nixon Peabody LLP, who counsels corporations, said that social media should be one of many tools used in recruitment, in order to cast a wide net for potential candidates. To the extent that employers conduct a social media background check, *it is better to have either a third party or a designated person within the company who does not make hiring decisions do the check, and only use publicly available information, not requesting passwords for social media accounts.*[51]

BEST PRACTICES FOR EMPLOYERS WHEN CONDUCTING ONLINE SOCIAL MEDIA SEARCHES

Here are recommendations for vetting employment candidates via social media:

Have a Policy. As with most compliance-related topics, a written policy is a must. The policy can be included in your practice's overall social media policy or it can be a stand-alone policy related only to the use of social media for hiring practices. Regardless, the policy should be clear as to who will be performing the searches.

It should also state the purpose of the search. Generally, the purpose is to validate information contained in a candidate's resume. Another purpose is to gain additional insight into the candidate's ability to perform job tasks. I recommend including in the policy a statement that your practice will only seek public information and will not attempt to trick, deceive, or coerce a candidate into revealing information on private social media accounts.

I pause here to say that I have had a client who viewed themselves as very clever by saying that it was not a requirement for a candidate to reveal social media platforms but merely a suggestion. Do not confuse clever with dangerous. This is not a thing to do. You need an all-out prohibition on accessing a candidate's private social media postings.

Finally, some policies limit the social media platforms the employer will review. If you are only going to look at Facebook and Instagram, then have your policy say so.

Be Consistent. Consistency is one of the keys to all compliance-related activities. Execute your policy the same way for each candidate. No one wants to face an argument that hiring practices are more thorough and rigorous for certain protected classes. Ralph Waldo Emerson famously stated that "…consistency is the hobgoblin of little minds." That may be. However, hobgoblins do not get sued.

Divide and Conquer. Use a two-prong approach when conducting social media searches. Have one person review the candidate's social media pages and posts pursuant to your practice's policy. However, to remove bias, have a second person be in charge of the actual hiring. This creates somewhat of an artificial wall between certain content that we do not want injected into the hiring process relative to the information that is legal and legitimate to use. This approach is a bit more time-consuming and slightly awkward. However, it does provide an extra layer of protection against claims of bias or discrimination.

Document. Make notes on the social media searches at the time they are performed. Notes do not need to be extensive but should show the searchers were compliant with the practice's policy. If questioned in the future, you want to be able to say, "Here are the notes on what we did and when we did it."

Color within the Lines. While most people know there are boundaries on the type of questions that can be asked of a job candidate, far fewer can properly describe those boundaries. Additionally, as we have seen, many states have specific laws regarding the use of social media when hiring. This all leads me to recommend you have a labor law attorney review your policies and procedures if there is any question in your mind as to whether some activity is permissible. What may seem creative or clever may actually turn out to be illegal. David St. Hubbins, a character from the movie "This is Spinal Tap," said it best: "It is such a fine line between stupid and clever." When in doubt, consult an expert.

SOCIAL MEDIA POLICIES FOR EMPLOYEES: THE ILLUSION OF CONTROL

In December 2009, Dawnmarrie Souza had a bad day. She was employed as an EMT for the American Medical Response Company that supplies ambulance service to many parts of the country. She apparently had inadequately filled out an incident report relating to a patient's complaint and as a result, was suspended by her supervisor. Souza disagreed with the supervisor's discipline strategy and took to Facebook. In what we can only imagine was a fit of pique, Souza posted "Looks like I am getting some time off. Love how the company allows a 17 to become a supervisor…" (A 17 was the company's terminology for a psychiatric patient.) But Souza wasn't done venting. In another post, she wrote that the supervisor was "being a dick" and was a "scumbag." Her comments did not go unnoticed. American Medical Response fired her shortly after the post went public[2,6].

American Medical Response's action was taken before the National Labor Relations board to determine if Souza's employment termination was proper. This case became one of the very first in which the National Labor Relations Board (NLRB) put the spotlight on what they believe to be unfair labor practices relating to employee use of social media.

The Souza matter alerted the public that NLRB applies to employees broadly in the private sector and that the NLRB was interested in pursuing charges against employers where social media policies or adverse employment actions have been alleged to have infringed on employees' protective activities.[7] Ultimately, Souza and American Medical Response arrived at a confidential settlement, but the case had ushered in a new era of oversight of social media policies.

The National Labor Relations Board is empowered by certain laws to protect employees from a variety of workplace harms, whether it is working conditions, pay, union organizing, or the ability to communicate on work-related topics. The NLRB has taken the position that modes of employee communication come under its jurisdiction, communication through social media will be treated the same as employee-created posters or handouts. Many will be surprised that even nonunion employees in the private sector are covered by the National Labor Relation Act, which is overseen by the NLRB. A full discussion of the history and scope of jurisdiction is beyond the scope of this book. Suffice to say the NLRB may be relevant to your practice.[7]

Practices need to be very careful when crafting a social media policy. The policy should not prohibit employees' discussion of working conditions or compensation even if those discussions are negative in nature. The case of *Hispanics United of Buffalo, Inc.*(359 N.L.R.B. no 37(2012) should serve as a cautionary tale. Hispanics United of Buffalo, Inc. is a nonprofit organization that assists victims of domestic violence. One of its employees, Lydia Cruz-Moore, felt that some of her coworkers were not performing up to standards. She sent a text to an unnamed co-worker complaining that she did more for victims than some of the other employees. This text message was ultimately shared with some of those coworkers being criticized. The criticized coworkers quickly took to Facebook with angry posts about Cruz-Moore's comment, such as "What the hell, we don't have a life as it is" and "Try doing my job. I have 5 programs."

The situation soon made its way to the Board of Directors of Hispanics United of Buffalo. The board felt that Cruz-Moore had been bullied and harassed by her fellow employees and that the actions were a violation of the nonprofit's "zero tolerance" policy. The board fired the employees involved in the Facebook exchange. But the story does not end there. The matter came to the attention of the NLRB, which determined employees had been improperly terminated. The NLRB ruled that the comments were for "mutual aid or protection" and came under Section 7 of the National Labor Relations Act. The employees were reinstated with back pay.

Another example comes from Swindon, a lovely town in England. There apparently are some cheeky individuals who work at Great Western Hospital in Swindon. These individuals included seven doctors and nurses who decided to play the "lying down" game on Facebook. For the uninitiated, this game is where a photograph is taken of an individual lying face down with their toes pointed to the floor. Extra credit is given to unusual posts or settings where these photographs were taken. The game on Facebook at one time had in excess of 70,000 members.

Well seven of our friends at Great Western Hospital became quite creative. Some were depicted on the helipad while some others were on gurneys or even the floor of the wards of the hospital. While all of this was done in good nature, the conduct was viewed as unprofessional by administrators of Great Western Hospital. The seven were suspended, but ultimately all went back to work at the hospital.

I include this example to show that social media issues faced by healthcare providers are not unique to the United States. More importantly, social media issues can arise without anyone violating patient privacy or being mean-spirited. Nonetheless, they have to be addressed.[8]

Not all employee comments that are negative in nature enjoy legal protection. Unfortunately, there are multiple examples of healthcare workers posting racists rants on social media, and social media policies have been used to discharge these employees. For example, an employee of Novant Health Presbyterian Center in Charlotte, North Carolina was terminated after she posted racists comments stating that black people where "dead weight on the American economy." She also posted "If I were a black female in America I would go live in the woods. I would be so ashamed of my race. To me it would be a curse to be black."[9]

Employee and social media policies that call for all patients to be treated with respect, fairness, and courtesy have been consistently upheld when challenged. I think that we can all agree that anyone that holds the racist opinions above does not need to be providing healthcare services.

As was previously mentioned, not all employment claims fall under federal law. When a Pennsylvania nurse was denied unemployment compensation benefits after being fired for using Facebook while at work, she took the matter to the Commonwealth Court of Pennsylvania. Here are the facts:

The nurse worked for Life Quest Nursing Center, which had a policy prohibiting the use of cellphones while on duty. The nurse had been made aware of this policy, yet she continued to make posts to Facebook using her cellphone. In fact, she used her cellphone to post comments on Facebook about a coworker who accidentally soiled her pants at work.

An investigation by Life Quest revealed that the nurse had been actively working (not on a break) at the time of the post. Further investigation revealed that the nurse was distributing medication to patients while the comments were posted. Life Quest discharged the nurse for engaging in conduct that could be life threatening and jeopardizing a patients' safety by using her cellphone and posting to Facebook while distributing patient medication.

The nurse sought unemployment benefits after being fired by Life Quest. Thankfully, the Unemployment Compensation Review Board determined that the nurse had engaged in willful misconducted and therefore should be ineligible for worker's compensation benefits. Undeterred, the nurse appealed the matter to the Commonwealth of Pennsylvania. The Commonwealth Court of Pennsylvania appealed the board's ruling and determined the nurse was not entitled to any employment compensation benefits.

The existence of the Life Quest cellphone policy was critical. The fact that the policy prohibited the behavior and that the employee was aware of the policy and the prohibition provided the necessary grounds to deny employment compensation benefits. This is a key point. We would all agree that posting a coworker accidentally soiling herself while distributing medication is inappropriate. Collectively we can scream "Outrageous!" However, this does not provide the sufficient legal structure to protect the practice. Policies are needed as is instruction on those policies. This is not the only case where a policy stemmed liability for a medical practice.[10]

Although we have focused on employees, a well-written and executed social media policy may prevent liability claims by patients as well. The University of Cincinnati Medical Center experienced this firsthand. A financial service staffer at University of Cincinnati Medical Center unfortunately shared a patient's syphilis diagnosis. This diagnosis was shared with the patient's ex-boyfriend. Things quickly took an ugly turn. Screen shots of the patient's medical records with diagnoses, taken by a hospital employee, were published on the Facebook page of a group called "Team No Hoes." As if this posting was not enough (and we certainly would all agree that it was), additional comments about the woman were also posted, labeling her a "slut" and a "hoe." The Facebook group had more than 2,200 members according to Facebook.[11]

As you might imagine, the patient sought legal counsel and filed a claim against not only the individuals involved in the posting but also the University of Cincinnati Medical Center.

In November 2015, an Ohio judge ruled that the University of Cincinnati Medical Center was not liable for the malicious actions of its employee. The court reasoned that the actions of the employee were outside the scope of her employment and that University of Cincinnati Medical Center's policy clearly prohibited the behavior in question of its employee. As a result of this ruling, the University of Cincinnati Medical Center was dropped from the litigation.[12] Here a well-crafted and utilized social media policy helped shield the University of Cincinnati Medical Center from liability for privacy breach.

Onslow Memorial Hospital is located in Jacksonville, North Carolina. It is a 162-bed facility with a staff of more than 100 physicians.[13] In May 2017, a mother and her two children were taken to Onslow after an automobile collision. The mother subsequently died. Working that day at Onslow was Olivia O'Leary, a medical technician. O'Leary saw a posting about the collision and the death of the mother. O'Leary posted "Should have worn her seatbelt…" O'Leary then went about her daily activities. Only later did she realize that the cyber community did not take kindly to her comment. O'Leary later claimed that she was trying to raise general awareness for seatbelts saving lives. Responding to an online thread, she also stated "Yep. I was working today when they came in the ER." According to a reporter interview given to a local news outlet, O'Leary stated she was fired for a patient privacy breach.[14]

The Onslow Memorial Hospital employee breach of patient privacy is typical of a category of social media patient privacy breaches. Here we did not have any malicious intent, no photographs or detailed medical information were posted, just an employee upset by the death of a mother making a few comments on social media after a hard day at work.

While completely understandable, this is impermissible. It is this type of situation that calls for a social media policy and instructions on that policy to keep a practice safe.

SOCIAL MEDIA STRATEGIES FOR LOWERING LIABILITY

For the safety of your medical practices, you need to have a social media strategy in place. Not only will proper policies and strategies protect your practice from employment discrimination claims, they also will protect you from third-party (including patients) liability claims. Here is what you should do:

1. Draft a comprehensive cellphone/mobile device policy as well as a comprehensive social media policy for your practice. Templates of both of these policies are included, in Section V, for your reference.
2. Make sure the social media policy and the cellphone/mobile device policy are reasonable, calculated to promote compliance and patient safety without being overly broad or restrictive. While it is appropriate to protect patient privacy and patient safety, it is

not appropriate or advisable to attempt to silence any complaint or critique associated with the management or operation of the medical practice.

3. Once policies are in place, the battle is only half won. Employees must be instructed on these policies. They must be accessible and used by your medical practice. You do not get any credit or bonus points for having nicely worded policies in a dusty three ring binder on your shelf.

4. In the event that a staff member violates social media policy or cellphone/mobile device policy, there needs to be consequence. I am not suggesting that the staff member be fired, but there must be some discipline as a result of a violation. A policy that is unenforced is either meaningless or arbitrary. Neither of these are good for your practice.

5. Finally, technology and social media change over time. This means that you need to revisit your policies on a routine basis. What is appropriate today may not be sufficient for a year from now. Add to your compliance calendar a future date to review the social media and cellphone/mobile device policies you are now implementing.

REFERENCES

1. Du W. Job candidates getting tripped up by Facebook, Nbcnews.com, August 14, 2007. http://www.nbcnews.com/id/20202935/ns/business-school_inc_/t/job-candidates-getting-tripped-facebook#.W6PegFJReV5. Accessed August 30, 2018.

2. Caers R and Castelyns V. LinkedIn and Facebook in Belgium. The influences and biases of social network sites in recruitment and selection procedures. *Social Science Computer Review* 29:437-48 (2011). https://www.researchgate.net/publication/258190136_LinkedIn_and_Facebook_in_Belgium_The_Influences_and_Biases_of_Social_Network_Sites_in_Recruitment_and_Selection_Procedures. Accessed August 30, 2018.

3. Seyfarth Shaw LLP. Social media privacy legislation. What employers need to know desktop reference, 2017–2018 Edition. Seyfarth Shaw LLP. www.seyfarth.com/uploads/siteFiles/practices/afabb55b685642048b41bc69f0acf51c_131317SocialMediaPrivacyLegislationDesktopReferenceM26.pdf. Accessed August 30, 2018.

4. McFarland S. & Valdes M. If you want a job, you may have to turn over your Facebook password. *Business Insider*. March 21, 2012. https://www.businessinsider.com/empoyers-ask-for-facebook-password-2012-3. Accessed August 30, 2018.

5. Equal Employment Opportunity Commission. Social media is part of today's workplace but its use may raise employment discrimination concerns. Press Release. March 12, 2014. https://www.eeoc.gov/eeoc/newsroom/release/3-12-14.cfm. Accessed August 30, 2018.

6. Kim S. NLRB backs worker fired after Facebook posts ripping boss. abcnews.go.com. November 10, 2010. https://abcnews.go.com/Business/facebook-firing-labor-board-takes-stand/story?id=12099395. Accessed August 30, 2018.

7. O'Brien C. The top 10 NLRB cases on Facebook firings and employer social media policies. 44 Acad. Legal Stud. In Bus. National Proc. Aug 2013. http://alsb.org/wp-content/uploads/2013/11/NP-2013-OBrien_Top-Ten-NLRB.pdf. Accessed August 30, 2018.

8. Fleming G. Hospital staff reinstated after 'lying down game' suspensions. The Nursing Times. October 14, 2009. https://www.nursingtimes.net/news/hospital/hospital-staff-reinstated-after-lying-down-game-suspensions/5007351.article. Accessed August 30, 2018.

9. Bleier K. Employee gone from hospital after posting racist comments on Facebook. *The Charlotte Observer*, July 14, 2016. https://www.charlotteobserver.com/news/local/article89551397.html. Acccessed August 30, 2018.

10. Meyer E. No unemployment benefits for woman fired for Facebooking at work. *The Employer Handbook Blog.* May 2, 2011. https://www.theemployerhandbook.com/no-unemployment-comp-for-woman. Accessed August 30, 2018.

11. Mottl J. Facebook posting on patient's diagnosis leads to hospital firing action. *Tech Times.* June 9, 2104. www.techtimes.com/articles/8204/20140609/facebook-posting-patients-diagnosis-leads-hospital-firing-action.htm. Accessed August 30, 2018.

12. WLWT5. Judge: UC Medical Center not liable after employee posted patient's record online. WWLWT5. com. November 10, 2015. www.wlwt.com/article/judge-cincinnati-hospital-not-liable-for-worker-s-facebook-post/3559738. Accessed August 30, 2018.

13. Onslow Memorial Hospital. About Us. www.onslow.org/about-us. Accessed August 30, 2018.

14. Thames A. OMH employee says she was fired over Facebook comment. *JDnews.* May 7, 2017. http://www.jdnews.com/news/20170507/omh-employee-says-she-was-fired-over-facebook-comment. Accessed August 30, 2018.

The Content You Create: Internal Risks and Management

1. LIABILITY.COM: DON'T LET YOUR WEBSITE TURN INTO A LAW SUIT

HOW TO MINIMIZE RISK AND IMPROVE COMPLIANCE

What could be more legally benign than a basic practice website?

You know the drill. You post some information about yourself that would make your mother proud. Add some facts about the staff, put up photos of the office, and finally, invite potential patients to "Contact Us." Much like a "glamour shot," it's intended to make you look as great as possible without crossing the line into fiction.

A medical practice website is straightforward, noncontroversial, and displays only the facts. Yours might be as outdated as a Motorola flip phone, but really, what could go wrong?

Sadly, plenty of things. Take what happened to a surgeon in south Texas as an example.

"Doctor, there's something you need to know," said the surgeon's patient, who found a website designed to look like the physician's but which clearly wasn't anything he would have approved for launch. The *About Us* section contained such statements as, "We recognize this may be a stressful time for you, so we'll do everything possible to maximize your pain and suffering." These statements were complemented by inflammatory fake posts that included such comments as "not so sudden death" and "deal with it, junkie."

Upon investigation, it was learned that the website had been active for several *months*. The surgeon immediately contacted the authorities, who traced the website back to a disgruntled patient who also happened to be an amateur web designer. Ultimately, he was arrested for felony online impersonation, but the reputational damage during the months this impostor website was active was already done. Unfortunately, this surgeon is not alone in experiencing real troubles from the virtual world.

This chapter provides guidance for reducing the risk that something like this can happen to your practice website. It offers strategies and tactics to help your practice:

- Choose a knowledgeable web developer that takes risk management seriously.
- Understand critical contract terms and negotiate a deal that protects you.
- Ensure that all data, images, and content are securely transmitted and stored.
- Develop and include the right disclosures, consents, and Terms of Use.
- Launch a site that is accessible to those with visual and hearing disabilities.

HACKING IS NOT LIMITED TO NETWORKS

Is it possible for a practice to be hacked through its website's *Contact Us* feature?

A few years ago, the Harley Medical Group in the UK learned that the answer is, *yes*. The aesthetic practice operates 21 clinics. It reported that information from approximately 480,000 patients and perspective patients was compromised through website hacking. Patient identities were "ransomed" back to the practice. Unlike most identity thieves who wish to use the information to obtain credit and goods, these hackers wanted to extort the practice. "Pay up or we will release your patients' information," they insisted.

This is only one example of "ransomware" being used to extort a medical practice. In fact, the FBI has recently issued warnings that this variety of cybercrime is on the rise.

If you really want to read something scary, put down the Stephen King novel and conduct a search on Google using the keywords *"Medical Website Hacked."* Searching these keywords yielded about 1,330,000 results in February 2018.[1] That's more than double the 607,000 results we got when we conducted the same search in May 2016. The results of the latest search included such headlines as "Fertility Clinic Hacked and Held for Ransom" and "Hacker Selling 655,000 Patient Records from 3 Hacked Healthcare Organizations."

Although these scenarios may seem dramatic, they have been plucked from real headlines. And as the increase in our search results illustrates, cyber wrongdoing and theft are on the rise. The number of healthcare data breaches has increased each year since 2015: from 270 that year to 327 in 2016 and 347 in 2017, according to the *HIPAA Journal*.[2] Add to that these facts: In 2017, 45% of all ransomware attacks were in the healthcare sector, and the largest occurrences in 2017 were due to hacking.[3]

This exponential growth shows no signs of abating, which means your practice must be vigilant. While it's virtually impossible to guarantee your site will not be hacked or control over it assumed by some rogue patient, there's no need to adopt the defeatist attitude that "no matter what I do, my website will never be secure." That's the medical equivalent of your patient saying, "Well doctor, I am going to die anyway so I might as well smoke three packs of cigarettes a day and stuff as much red meat down my gullet as possible." Rest assured, there are actions you can take to minimize the risk.

CENTS AND SENSIBILITY

Most physicians think of their website as a marketing expense. And as any smart businessperson hopes to do, they want to spend as little as possible on it.

If you've started down the road of evaluating website developers, you know that their proposals can come in at $10,000 or more. So, to save money, you might be considering building the site yourself by taking your own photos, writing the copy, and using low-cost site building tools such Wordpress or Square Space. Let me disabuse you of this plan. Thinking you will save money by doing it yourself (DIY) is a bad idea. The reason is simple: *you don't know what you don't know.* And that means you won't know what you have overlooked. It would be like me attempting to save money by repairing my own car, even though the truth is, I don't know anything about cars. When I hear a noise under the hood, I don't know if it's the alternator belt or the serpentine belt. That's why it's in my own best interest (and safety) to take it to a professional instead of looking under the hood to figure out the problem on my own.

So, although you might think that using Wordpress is an easy way to launch a DIY site, low-cost tools such as this one are not intended for use by healthcare organizations without significant customization and additional programming. In fact, "out of the box," these tools often lack essential HIPAA requirements such as email transmission encryption, storage, backup encryption, and integrity validation (meaning that there is no way to determine if data on your site has been tampered with).

Wordpress in particular is notorious for being hacked, according to Brad Garnett, digital forensic examiner with Kemper Technology Consulting in Evansville, Indiana. He points out that, if you've ever built a Wordpress site, you know that to access the administrative panel, you go to www.yourdomain.com/*wp-admin*. Add to that the high percentage of folks who use "password" as their password, and it's not hard to understand why cyber thieves prefer to hack Wordpress sites. According to Garnett, most site owners leave the door wide open for them to easily do so.

Plus, you'd be hard-pressed to get these DIY web service providers to sign a Business Associate Agreement (BAA), which makes your practice out of compliance with HIPAA before the site even launches. (More on that shortly.)

Finally, let's not forget that you already have an overly packed patient schedule. Spending dozens (and in some cases hundreds) of hours getting a website off the ground is not a good use of your clinical skills. You wouldn't ask a website designer to diagnose and treat a suspicious lump on your neck. Don't attempt to plan, design, build, and maintain your own professional website. Even if you are a Millennial generation physician or someone who enjoys tinkering with software, healthcare website design and maintenance is a complex and nuanced industry. Again, *you won't know what you don't know.*

Before you build and launch something that causes you professional embarrassment or results in a lawsuit, give up the DIY route and seek professional assistance. Leave your website development and maintenance to someone whose full-time job it is to stay abreast of the technology, liability, and design issues required.

Now that we have escorted that elephant out of the room, let's focus on identifying a qualified and credible company to build and maintain your site.

WHERE OH WHERE CAN I FIND A GOOD WEB DEVELOPER?

"I have the perfect guy for you. He put together the website for our church."

"My neighbor's son's friend just graduated from State and started a web company. She is looking for clients so I'll bet you could hire her on the cheap."

These are a couple of the common responses you'll hear if you start telling friends and family that you are looking for a website designer. There are a lot of people out there who build websites. Many are excellent graphic designers and use tools that will make your site look very modern. But there are two important things for a physician to keep in mind:

1. A physician practice website requires more than just great design and graphics. Security, encryption, and compliance are essential.
2. You are entrusting your entire professional reputation to the company you choose.

Sure, your website is a marketing asset. But remember that it's also a source of potential liability. The content and links on your website need to comport with your state board of medicine's requirements. HIPAA, copyright, and trademark violations, lack of encryption and security, and failure to make the site accessible for those who have visual or hearing impairments are just a few of areas that physicians often don't think about when they are in the throes of designing a site.

Before you say yes to your sister's friend's daughter, use an objective screening and evaluation process to determine if she is indeed qualified. The last thing you want to do is trust your website to someone whom you wouldn't hire to feed the cat while you are away. Although the designer's sample sites might be appealing and the company may indeed use the slickest new design tools, if he or she has little to no knowledge of healthcare, a physician practice's online needs, ethical requirements, or HIPAA, you are putting your practice at risk.

And I can almost guarantee you that the newly minted college grad working from his spare bedroom won't know a BAA from a BLT (bacon, lettuce, and tomato). Avoid being someone else's learning curve.

According to Robert Baxter, CEO of Surgeon's Advisor, a provider of Internet marketing and patient acquisition strategies for aesthetic physicians, the simplest way to find a quality vendor is to ask colleagues for references and then review sites built by these companies to see what they look like and how they "feel" to you. The truth is, there is no "best" web-development company because site design is subjective. What you think is a great site may not resonate with someone else. To*may*to, to*mah*to, as it were. The important thing is that the site is right for you and your practice. That means you must feel comfortable with the web developer's design capabilities as well as its knowledge and management of security.

Here's how to start the evaluation process:

1. **Visit the sites of colleagues, competitors, and other physicians.** What have these physicians included on their sites? What do you like about them? What do you *not* like about them? Keep a log of your findings—they will be useful as you talk with designers. On the sites you like, look at the bottom to see if the developer's name is listed and contact them. Or, contact the physician and ask who they used.
2. **Get a referral from professional advisors you trust.** Your accountant, attorney, or marketing and public relations firms probably work with other physicians and may know of web-development firms they have used.
3. **Contact your practice management system vendor.** If the vendor offers a physician portal, it may also provide website services. Keep in mind that if you want a fully custom site, this option may not be the ideal fit, as these vendors typically provide sites based on templates and the sites can look somewhat "cookie cutter." But for some physicians, the template approach may be just fine, and the price tag is often much lower than a custom site.

4. **Ask friends who work in other business industries.** If you trust their business acumen, you can probably trust their referral.

Do your homework on each of the companies referred your way. Stop, look, and review in detail their site portfolios so you have a good sense about their design skills. Don't contact them before you know that the look and feel of their work is what you are looking for.

For those companies that pass your design "sniff test," screen their site portfolios as well as their company website for these critical characteristics:

1. *Does the developer build websites for physicians and/or hospitals?* Be leery about companies that have never built a site for a physician practice, a hospital, or another Covered Entity. There's a high chance the company will not effectively build a site that complies with HIPAA requirements and it's likely they've never signed a BAA. Likewise, if a firm has no experience building an accessible site or a responsive design site, they are not the choice for your practice.

2. *If you practice in a niche or elective specialty, does the company work in your specialty?* If you are an internist this probably is not so important. But if you are in a specialty such as cosmetic surgery, Lasik, or cosmetic dermatology, a specialty web-development firm is advisable. Baxter's company deals exclusively with aesthetic practices, allowing them to understand that specialty's needs at a very deep level. Niche specialties have an elective, private pay element to at least some of the procedures performed. The patients they treat typically have higher standards for service and marketing, and a web developer that offers lead generation and search engine optimization (SEO) are necessary.

3. *Does the company promote its experience with maintaining privacy, security, or understanding HIPAA?* Look for language on their website as evidence of this.

4. *Does the company's "About Us" page include people you can imagine yourself working with?* You will be spending a lot of time with these folks as you develop the site. And they'll probably maintain the site as well. Make sure the working relationship is a potential fit. It does not matter how skilled and knowledgeable the company is if the people annoy you or aren't your style.

Finally, what if you already have a fantastic web developer you trust and find to be reliable? That's great but remember to read the information about contract terms and BAAs that follows, to make sure this vendor relationship is safe and compliant.

CONDUCT A RISK ASSESSMENT WITH VENDORS

My destiny as an attorney could probably have been predicted based on how many questions I asked as a kid. I was that impossibly curious child who always sat in the front row and asked a lot of questions. Doing so gave me a much better understanding of the topic we were studying.

Although these days my curiosity can occasionally annoy my teenage sons, asking questions serves me well as I evaluate contracts and documents and assess the HIPAA compliance of physician practices. And I recommend this question-driven approach to clients when it comes to evaluating vendors.

There are seven, high-priority questions to ask the final two or three contenders for your website business. The questions, their rationale, and some of the possible correct answers are shown below. Included in the Appendix at the end of this chapter is a comprehensive list of website designer questions. But if you are short on time, at least ask these seven, which indicate the vendor's knowledge of healthcare privacy and security risk.

High-Priority Questions to Ask a Website Designer

1. *Who purchases/owns the domain?* You should be the only one to purchase the domain. It's a red flag if the vendor offers to do this for you.
2. *Who owns the content on the website?* Again, the answer must be *you*. Except for stock images the vendor may suggest licensing, you should own all content on the site. And this must clear in the written contract.
3. *What do you do within your company to comply with HIPAA?* This one will separate the wheat from the chaff. The vendor should be able to describe pretty much the same things that your practice has done to comply with HIPAA, because the HIPAA Omnibus Rule requires all business associates to comply in the same way that Covered Providers do. Answers could include: require initial and annual HIPAA training for all employees and independent contractors; use secure, encrypted email when sending ePHI; or maintain a breach policy.
4. *How do you ensure that all of our content and images, as well as any data from site visitors, is stored and transferred securely?* The answer is that the vendor will establish secure connections to encrypt any information submitted on the site (such as through a Contact Us form or to request an appointment), as well as between servers as content and images are posted to the site. This kind of "transport encryption" is required by HIPAA and is best accomplished by obtaining Secure Sockets Layer (SSL) certificates, which ensure the secure point-to-point transmission of content. A more detailed explanation of why your practice should purchase these is shown in Figure III-1.
5. *Tell me what you do to ensure accessibility? Which guidelines do you follow?* The vendor should know about the WC3 guidelines for web accessibility. (More about this at the end of this chapter.) They should know about how visually and hearing-impaired people use devices to "read" the site. They might share specific ways they comply with accessibility, such as adding contextual text to all images, offering multiple font sizes, or creating clear content headers on all pages so devices can easily read them.
6. *If we decide to part ways, in what format do you deliver all of our content and images and what is the process for doing so?* The answer should include the process for uploading your data via a secure connection.
7. *Do you have cyber insurance that covers us both while we are working together?* Breaches are very expensive and, sadly, common. Your website vendor needs to have appropriate cyber insurance coverage in the event of an attack. Beyond the security that comes with the coverage, this is a good litmus test of the vendor's focus on safety and professionalism.

FIGURE III-1. In God We Trust—All Others Need SSL Certificates

SSL (Secure Sockets Layer) certificates, also known as digital certificates, are security protocols that facilitate encrypted communication between a web server and a web browser. They are used to reduce the risk of sensitive data such as protected health information (PHI) being intercepted and stolen while it's being transmitted between a person's browser and a server on the Internet. You can tell when a connection is certified because the web address displays "https" instead of "http." The process of digitally certifying the connection creates a "secure pipe" through which information can travel from one place to another online, without nefarious hackers being able to grab it.

SSL certificates are purchased from a Certificate Authority—a company that authenticates the identity of a website and encrypts the data travelling through the pipe. SSL certificates cost very little and can provide great peace of mind for your practice. A web developer can assist you in obtaining SSL certificates or you can purchase them from your domain name registrar. Best practice is to obtain *a certificate for every online connection point* between all servers and software applications used over the Internet. This includes, but is not limited to, the connections between practice computers and the website host, practice computers and the content management system (CMS), and the web developer's computers and any website testing servers used during development.

CONTRACT TERMS

You found three or four reputable vendors whose website portfolios impressed you. Two made it through the risk assessment interrogation. After checking references and reviewing the price of the proposal, you chose a final vendor. Congratulations, you're ready to go to contract.

The contract is the document that establishes responsibilities for both your practice and the web developer so everyone is clear and has the same expectations. Even more important, it protects you from certain liabilities. Engage an attorney to review it and point out issues of concern. Skipping this step is pennywise and pound-foolish.

Several years ago, I had a client who asked me review a proposed contract from a website developer. The contract had terms that claimed the developer made no warranties that the site would function and a clause that gave the website developer full immunity. Needless to say, these provisions did not match what the salesmen had told my client. Ultimately, the contract was cleaned up, but it could have been a big problem. When contracting with a website vendor, operate under the mode of "trust but verify."

Here are the major areas to be concerned with:

1. *Domain Ownership.* Domain names are inexpensive to purchase but can cost you a lot if the wrong person owns them. I've reviewed many contracts that essentially say that the web developer will purchase and maintain the domain on your behalf. *Change this before you sign.* You must purchase the domain in your own name. Never agree to a contract that allows a web developer to buy your domain. It's akin to giving them the keys to the kingdom.

   Purchase the domain not only for your personal name and practice name, but other closely related derivatives as well. For example, I want to control not just "Sacopulos.com," but also "Sacopulos Law Firm.com" and "Sacopulos Sucks.com" (You can never be too careful).

2. *Content Ownership.* The content owner should always be the physician or the practice, and that must be clearly stated in the contract. Make sure it reads that you own all forms of content, including text, images, patient photos, and data.

3. *Copyrights.* If you own the content and images on the website, the copyrights should be yours or those of the practice. Be sure this is explicit in the contract so the web developer has no opportunity to assume the copyrights themselves. In addition, this section should cover content and images whose copyrights are owned by others, stating that your web developer agrees never to post anything to the site without direct permission from the owner.

4. *Patient Images.* The only patient images that should be on the website are those that are owned by the physician or the practice.

5. *Americans with Disabilities Act (ADA) Compliance.* Often there is a boilerplate con-tract item that says something like, "We agree to follow all state and federal regula-tions, as required by law." With ADA, you want more specificity in the contract. A clause should say that the web developer will develop an accessible site that follows the recommended guidelines from WC3.

6. *HIPAA Compliance.* The contractual elements for HIPAA should be covered in a BAA. If the vendor has never signed one, or has never heard of such a document, that's a red flag—although not necessarily a deal breaker if the vendor has checked out on all other evaluation points. Refer to the section in this chapter about BAAs for the detailed components related to HIPAA compliance.

7. *Insurance Coverage.* Your concern should be twofold: First, does the web developer carry liability insurance? Second, is the amount sufficient to cover a breach if, in the post-launch maintenance phase, the site is hacked and patient info is taken? The amount of insurance coverage the vendor should have depends on the needs of your practice. Because this varies widely, contact your own insurance broker and ask for a free estimate. Ask him or her how much liability coverage you have currently and what amount he or she believes is appropriate for a vendor to have, given your busi-ness goals.

8. *Time Commitments and "Who Does What?"* This is the opportunity to discuss and clarify with the vendor things such as: Who is writing the content? Where will you get the images? What are the timelines, deadlines, and testing processes? How many hours per week does the vendor estimate will be required by your manager to write, or test, or coordinate?

   Go into the relationship with your eyes wide open. If the vendor plans to slough off coordination tasks, or copyediting, or certain testing elements, you need to know that in advance. Participating in these duties during development may temporarily take staff away from their primary job with patients, billing, or management. Plan accordingly.

9. *Breakup Process.* Ask for written details. Do you have to give a certain number of days' notice to avoid fines? How will content be delivered back to the practice? Electronically or on digital devices? How quickly will the vendor respond when you want to close up shop with them?

10. *Don't Share My Stuff.* Some vendors monitor the traffic and/or the improvement of lead generation on their client sites and use this in marketing and sales to others. Although this is a valid use of business information for demonstrating the web developer's value to potential customers, I still recommend to physicians that they disallow web developers to use the client's data for this purpose. The last thing you want when vendors are pitching themselves to your competitors, or someone in your same specialty, is for them to say things such as "We increased patient leads for Dr. *Your Name Here* by 40%." Your contract should state that whatever quantitative or qualitative data the vendor collects and/or has access to about your site or its activity is not to be shared with anyone except authorized individuals in your practice.

THE BUSINESS ASSOCIATE AGREEMENT (BAA)

Unless you have been practicing under a rock, you know that the HIPAA Omnibus Rule requires all business associates, no matter how big or small, to follow the same rules your practice does when it comes to the privacy and security of protected health information (PHI). That means if a web developer does not have a breach policy and procedure, or does not provide initial and annual HIPAA training to its employees and independent contractors who work on your website, or does not use a web host that is HIPAA compliant, technically speaking, your practice is not HIPAA compliant.

If you haven't updated your BAA in recent memory, contact a healthcare attorney to ensure it meets all of the HIPAA Omnibus Rule requirements. In contractual relationships such as the one with a web developer, I frequently find that physicians have not asked the vendor to sign a BAA, or the one that has been signed is outdated. The BAA protects the privacy of your patients and ultimately the reputation of your practice.

To comply with HIPAA, your BAA must include these seven essential clauses, and the web developer must demonstrate they can deliver on each one.

1. Indemnification clause. This holds your practice harmless from any untoward event related to the website or patient data, should that untoward event be caused by the vendor.
2. General liability (GL) and errors and omissions (E&O) insurance coverage, each with a coverage limit of at least $1 million.
3. Breach notification procedure. Ask to see the procedure to verify that it exists.
4. Data security policy. Ask to see the procedure to verify that it exists.
5. Privacy policy.
6. Secure communication/transmission of data and PHI to/from website forms and between servers used to store content and images.
7. Procedure for returning all of your content, images, and other data to the practice at the termination of the agreement and destroying all incidences of digital and paper

records. This clause should also include the procedure for disabling company access to your content management system and website host.

DISCLOSURES, CONSENTS, AND TERMS ... *OH MY*

If I call most medical practices at 9 p.m. on a Friday, I'll get an answering machine. The message will tell me the practice's hours and instruct me to dial 911 if I'm having a medical emergency.

However, if I access the same practice's website at 9 p.m. on Friday via the *Contact Us* page, I most likely will not receive that same instruction to 911 if I am experiencing a medical emergency.

Let's set aside the fact that a patient who is having a heart attack and believes contacting a physician through his or her website page for help probably lacks good judgment. That is a topic for a different chapter, perhaps one about abnormal psychology. The point is that, like the outgoing message on your voice mail, the *Contact Us* page must warn the patient about what to do if he or she is experiencing an emergency. Although this disclosure may seem to clinicians as obviously necessary, it is important to the practice's online liability management.

In addition, there are several other important disclosures to put on a practice website, each of which can reduce liability and risk. Work with a healthcare attorney to make sure the language you post follows the laws in your state.

On the *Contact Us* page:

1. *If this is a medical emergency, please call 911 immediately.* You might also add: "Our practice does not handle emergencies through this website."
2. *You aren't a patient if you don't have a medical record on file.* Sample language: "Submitting information via this page (or form) does not create a patient/physician relationship. You are not a patient of [Practice Name] unless you have been seen by one of our physicians and have a medical chart on file with our office."
3. *Information submitted is not encrypted or secure.* Although the HIPAA Omnibus Rule does require providers to encrypt the transmission of ePHI of data "at rest" (for instance, to and from a database or from server to server), such a requirement does not exist for data "in transmission." Physicians still, however, have a duty to advise patients and potential patients not to send certain personal and medical information through a website form. The *Contact Us* page should have a disclosure such as: "This is not a secure or encrypted means of communicating with our practice. Do not enter your social security number, date of birth, or other medical information on this form."

On a *Blog* page:

Not a substitute for medical advice. Many clinicians write blogs that provide general medical information or discuss topics that they think may be relevant to their patients. If you are one of them, post a disclosure associated with the blog saying, "This information is *not* meant as medical advice. It is provided solely for education. Our practice would be pleased to discuss your unique circumstances and needs as they relate to these topics." Although a blog is not a tremendous area of risk, a simple disclosure may be helpful.

For the *Terms of Use*:

Terms of Use govern the access and use of the website by visitors. It's not a requirement that all visitors to your website click to indicate they have read and accepted them, but from a risk management standpoint, it's important to develop and post these terms on the site. Commonly, practices provide a hyperlink on the bottom of all pages in the site and label it, *Terms of Use.* Interested website visitors can click on the link to read the page that displays this document.

A thorough *Terms of Use* typically includes:

- Copyright notices.
- Rules around the use of any intellectual property and/or images on the site.
- Privacy policy.
- A statement that the content on the site is not intended as medical advice.
- Limited liability statements that protect the practice against frivolous lawsuits.
- Indemnification language so that your practice is held harmless against any damages or actions taken as a result of someone visiting the site.

For *Consents:*

1. *Fine-tune your patient photo release.* A sample has been provided in Section V.
2. *Develop a general photo release, if you don't already have one.* If you take photographs during patient education events or seminars, ask all attendees to sign a general release. The disclosure should state that your practice owns the copyright to the image. This provides the documentation you would need if the photos on the site are ever "scraped." See Figure III-2 for more detail about "scraping."
3. *Obtain written authorization to use patient quotes and testimonials.* Both are an excellent way to convey your skills and service delivery from the patient's perspective. But you must have each patient's written permission before you post them to the website. In addition, make sure your state medical society's professional responsibility or conduct requirements allow you to use patient testimonials in your marketing efforts. Some states do not. Make sure yours is not one of them.

With regard to the images you did not create yourself, or for which your practice does **not** own the copyright, the practice must obtain a license or permission to use them. **Copying photos from another website or taking an image from Google Images is not legal.**

Some web designers search Google or scour the Internet for images and place them on their client sites. This is a big no-no. Firms such as Getty Images do indeed pursue (and charge a fee to) website owners who use their images without permission. The copyright laws are decidedly stacked against you and you will pay (or else!) if there is an image on your website that you don't have permission to use.

To stay out of legal trouble, purchase a subscription to an image site such as ThinkStock. com, and follow their rules for usage. Usually there is a small fee for the use of each image used. Cost-free and royalty-free image sites such as Unsplash.com are also an option.

FIGURE III-2. Protect Patient Photos Against "Scraping"

"It was both surprising and disturbing," said Seattle based attorney Greg Wesner of Lane Powell PC, when he recounted the story of representing a prominent West Coast-based facial plastic surgeon. His clients' before and after photographs were found on no fewer than 13 other medical practices websites around the country. "I don't know if it was the medical practices or their web designers who stole my clients' images," says Wesner. "What I do know is that it is legally actionable and we have been successfully going after the practices that display my clients' work as though it was their own."

Wesner's practice is not alone, I am aware of many practices that have faced similar situations. Even if you are not concerned images on your website will be "scraped" and used by others without your permission, you still need to be concerned about this issue.

Ask all patients whose photos you wish to use to sign a consent form. In addition to the form stating that the patient grants his or her permission for you to use the photos on the website and other communication efforts, it should state that your practice owns the copyright to the image because the physician or someone on the staff is the individual who took the photograph.

WEBSITE CONTENT AND THE ROLE OF THE FEDERATION OF STATE MEDICAL BOARDS

The Federation of State Medical Boards (FSMB) has issued guidance for physician use of the worldwide web and social media. Given its scope, it impacts web content too.

Section 4 of the Model Policy Guidelines specifically addresses posting content, stating: *"When posting content online, [physicians] should always remember that they are representing the medical community. Physicians should always act professionally and take caution not to post information that is ambiguous or could be misconstrued or taken out of context. Physician employees of healthcare institutions should be aware that employers reserve the right to edit, modify, delete, or review internet communications. **Physician writers assume all risks related to security, privacy and confidentiality of their posts.**"*

That last sentence must be considered if you are outsourcing content development for your website. You are on the hook for what is being posted under your name. If you engage a vendor to create or post content on behalf of the practice, make sure the company understands your ethical duties under the FSMB's guidelines If the vendor does not follow them, it may impact your professional reputation. In fact, over the past several years, a number of FSMB members have disciplined physicians for inappropriate online behavior.

And, there's even more you need to know about board guidance: Individual state boards of medicine have ethics rules that apply to a practice's website, too. Many of them are holdovers from the pre-digital age. From example, some states prohibit physicians from using patient testimonials. Other states do not allow the posting of before and after photographs, even with patient consent. Certain states prohibit the use of the generic term, "board certified," requiring that you provide the name of the specific board that has certified you.

Given the patchwork of obscure and anachronistic state boards of medicine's rules that apply to website content, consult your licensing board for specific guidance.

SITE SECURITY, HIPAA COMPLIANCE, AND YOU

I'm going to make the assumption that the majority of readers want their practice website to include a Contact Us form, a registration form, and a way for patients to request or make an appointment. You may choose to use a patient portal for some of these activities, but at the very least, your website should have a Contact Us form.

The truth is if you offer *any one of the above features*, your site is under the purview of HIPAA. And once you are in, there is no way out. So, let's discuss the intersection of site security and HIPAA compliance.

It behooves any industry to step up their website security, in order to avoid cyberthieves and hackers from stealing data, content, or intellectual property. Healthcare is no different, and the information that is of the highest priority to protect is the PHI of patients.

I'm going to again reference digital forensic examiner Brad Garnett, who says that the first order of business when securing a website is to think of the site as a house. (Gives new meaning to the term "home page," doesn't it?) A house has windows and it has doors, each of which presumably has a lock. The more windows and doors you leave unlocked when you head off the barber or the beach, the more opportunity there is for an unsavory character to enter the house and make off with the heirloom jewels you inherited from your Aunt Beatrice. Do a good job reminding the kids to lock up the place before they leave and you'll reduce the opportunity and threat of a break-in. Add an alarm system and you secure the house even more.

Garnett is quick to point out that many practices, and other businesses, frequently leave their digital front door unlocked—and often a couple of digital windows open too. Many security breaches, he contends, could have been avoided had the victimized organizations taken a few straightforward preventive steps. In addition to following the HIPAA requirements we have already covered, such as storing data on a secure, encrypted server and encrypting all data during transmission from servers or forms, Garnett suggests these tips:

1. *Keep all website code up to date.* Consider the last time your site was updated. If it's been five years or more, or the site was built on old versions of HTML or PHP, the code is more vulnerable to attack. Anyone can "right-click" on a web page and open up a window that displays all the code behind the page, as well as information about the site's structure and host severs.

   Garnett explains the risk like this: When a hacker sees that your code is outdated, he could potentially execute a cross-site scripting attack, embedding malicious code into yours that redirects data onto a fake site or a site that he maintains. From there, the data can be manipulated, sold, or used for identity theft. So, keeping the site code up to date and maintaining the newest programming libraries is like keeping the windows of your house closed and locked.

2. *Insist that your web developer use the most current versions of all software tools.* Most do. Some do not. Make sure your vendor is in the former camp. Not keeping up with the latest versions can result in old code being written into your website. (Refer to security tip #1.)

3. *Limit the number of web forms you offer on the site.* Forms are like windows: The more of them you have open the better chance dust will blow in. It's best to limit the site to having one or two forms and collect minimal PHI.

4. *Use a "Captcha" on the Contact Us form.* "Captcha" is that annoying little box that forces you to enter a series of letters or numbers that verify you are a real human, not a web bot. The idea is that you want only actual humans accessing your website, not computers. If your eyes are as good as mine, you have to ask it for at last five different combinations before you enter one accurately. That said, "Captcha" is a low-cost and simple way to add security to the communication channel used by the form.

5. *Include disclosures on the site, and especially on forms.* We've covered disclosures in general. Specific to maintaining security, Garnett suggests warning patients against entering sensitive data, such as a date of birth, into any form fields. A disclosure statement should precede any text field into which a visitor can provide unstructured information they feel is relevant, so he or she is reminded that entering personal or sensitive information is risky.

6. *Secure the link from the website to the patient portal, if you offer one.*

In addition to these precautionary steps, there is also one that you can take with your staff. Train them to be on alert for social engineering scams. Hackers and cyberthieves can obtain access to your online data by calling or emailing your practice, pretending to be a representative from say, your website hosting company, and asking your staff to provide login credentials for reasons such as "updating your information." Amazingly, many employees provide the information asked for. In fact, the majority of security breaches are the result of human error and not a flaw in software construction. Basic cyber hygiene training is absolutely critical to the safety of your patients' data. Figure III-3 provides tips for avoiding these social engineering scams.

SPECIALTY VENDORS REQUESTING ACCESS TO YOUR WEBSITE

Let me add a cautionary tale from several client practices that gave out the User ID and password to the back end of their website to a non-web developer vendor. The vendor requested these "keys to the kingdom," citing the convenience of posting their logo and a link to their website so the busy practice manager wouldn't have to. In each of the practices that provided the "keys," the logo of a competing vendor mysteriously vanished without the practice's permission.

The moral of this story is: except for your web vendor, never give this level of access to anyone outside of your practice—especially a vendor. There is no telling what can come of this level of access, but in my experience, it's often not good.

One consequence of distributing access information to your website is that it could void your cyber insurance policy. Some policies exclude breaches that arise from distribution of a password to a third-party vendor. Having gone to the effort and expense to secure cyber coverage, you might be undoing your good work by having the vendor "tweak" the website for you.

Peter Reilly, area executive vice president of healthcare of Arthur J. Gallagher & Co., is an expert on healthcare cyber insurance coverage. According to Reilly, "You certainly invite coverage concerns or claim payment problems when you have not taken the necessary precautions to protect your data and access to your website."

This means that distributing the password to your practice's website to third parties may have cyber insurance coverage implications. As Reilly explains, "You make warranties to the insurance company that you are taking certain steps to protect that information, so if you are willing to give out your password or other security measures to a third-party vendor, you put your coverage at risk because you are therefore willingly and intentionally opening the door to a potential claim." Reilly goes on to say that practices potentially put themselves at risk by not knowing a third-party vendor's IT security and cyber hygiene when handing over access to that website. Reilly recommends that in most instances, practices should not provide third-party vendors access to their website.

FIGURE III-3. How to Avoid a Social Engineering Scam

"Good morning, Dr. Caring's office, this is Sue. How may I help you?"

"Hi Sue, this is John from GoDaddy. We host your website domain and I'm calling to verify your login information for our files. Can you help me, please?"

"Sure! I check our web email daily so I have that information. What do you need?"

"I need to verify your User ID and password, the one you use to log into your hosting company. Do you have that?"

"Yes, hold on...Here it is, John. Our User ID is drcaringMD, and the password is Password123..."

You probably already guessed that John does not work for GoDaddy. John has just conned Sue out of the practice's login credentials. Most likely, John researched the practice's domain on a public site such as Whois.com and noticed GoDaddy as the host of the website. With this information, and probably a bit of charm, he was able to make Sue believe he was a good guy updating information, not a bad guy hoping to hack in and steal data. Attempting to be helpful, Sue played right into his hand, giving John full access to the back end of the practice's website.

This devious activity is form of *social engineering*, and you need to train your staff to be on the lookout for it. According to Wikipedia, social engineering, in the context of information security, refers to psychological manipulation of people into performing actions or divulging confidential information.[4]

Make your staff aware of the risks involved when they give out login credentials to your website, social media, or any online application. Train them to follow these guidelines:

1. Never provide User IDs or passwords to someone who calls the practice or sends an email. No one who calls *in* should ever be provided an ID or password. *Period.*
2. Never write IDs or passwords on a Post-It® or other obvious pieces of paper and leave them in plain view at the front desk. Devious hackers can easily see them—they know what they are looking for.
3. Tell staff to alert you or the practice manager if someone has contacted the practice and recommended this information.
4. Spend a few bucks each year to make your domain information private. Contact the company that hosts your domain to obtain pricing. Often this is the same company that hosts the website. Once you've made your domain information private, it will not be listed when someone searches for the owner of your domain. Social engineers cannot use information they cannot see.

ACCESSIBILITY FOR ALL

It comes as a surprise to many practices that their website must be compliant with the Americans with Disabilities Act (ADA). Under Title II of the act, all "places of public accommodations" cannot exclude those with disabilities from what is offered to everyone else. Every company that has a public website is obligated to comply, and that includes medical practices, no matter the number of employees or size of the practice.

The need for websites to be compliant with the ADA is not new. In fact, all United States federal websites have been compliant with the act for more than a decade. But over the last several years, there has been a new wave of litigation fueling the move toward website accessibility.

If you aren't familiar with the term, *accessibility* means for example, that the text on a website is written and constructed on a page in such a way that a visually impaired person can convert it into audio as the cursor moves across the screen, using a reading device. Or, that all videos on the site have closed-caption subtitles to enable a hearing-impaired person to read along while watching the video images. Or, that the site's font size can be made bigger or smaller to make it easier for senior eyes to read without straining. If the website has an audio component, closed captioning must be available for the hearing-impaired. Additionally, if you offer an employment application on your website, it must be able to be completed by someone who is disabled as well as someone who is not.

The National Federation of the Blind has brought class action lawsuits against a number of retailers for website non-compliance with the ADA. The organization sued Target, alleging that Target's website was not accessible to blind customers. Ultimately, the class action settled for multi-millions of dollars.

Individuals have also brought these types of lawsuits. A blind mother of three filed a claim against the Seattle Public Schools alleging the Seattle Public Schools website software was not compatible with a screen reading device.

As long as making a website accessible is not an undue burden, a company must provide access to the same information, services, and opportunity to participate to *everyone*. Generally speaking, a website that is not accessible denies a person the "opportunity to participate." So, for instance, if your website provides a series of educational videos for pre- and post-operative care, and they do not have closed captions, your website is not accessible. Fines for non-compliance can be as high as $75K for each incidence.

The good news is, there are many ways to make your website more accessible, and most of them cost little or nothing. The key is to be aware of them and direct your web developer to follow appropriate guidelines for implementing them on your site.

The best thing a practice and its web developer can do is to follow the Web Content Accessibility Guidelines (WCAG 2.0), available from W3C at https://www.w3.org/TR/WCAG20. W3C is a non-profit, international community where member organizations work together to develop web standards.

The WCAG 2.0 standards include design guidelines such as:[5]

- *Provide informative, unique page titles* and *use headings to convey meaning and structure.* These two guidelines make it easier for reader tools to find and interpret the text.
- *Use headings and spacing to group related content.* This allows "reader" devices to more easily locate and "read" to a visually impaired site visitor.
- *Write meaningful text alternatives to images.* If a web designer doesn't add text to describe each image on your site, a visually impaired person cannot "see" them using a reading device.
- *Make link text meaningful.* Descriptive text helps sight-impaired individuals discern what the link they are about to click on is linking them to.
- *Create designs for different viewport sizes.* When visitors opt to resize the text font, the design size remains relative to the text size.

Some accessibility advocates are calling the recent push toward accessibility "the new Civil Rights Movement." The ADA's intent is to make all websites accessible for those who are visually or hearing-impaired, or who have other disabilities that result in them not being able to access information on the Internet without a device or other means. The greater purpose here is to enable people with disabilities to participate in American life, much of which today occurs on the Internet.

CONCLUSION

Like many things in life, your website is not a problem until it is a problem. An ounce of prevention could save you from losing a pound of flesh. Now that you understand the liability issues associated with your practice website, use the tools and suggestions from this chapter to make sure your site doesn't turn into a law suit any time soon.

CHAPTER APPENDIX

- Risk Assessment Questions for Web Developers
- Liability.com Checklist

Risk Assessment Questions for Web Developers

Ask These Questions	Hope to Hear These Answers
1. Who purchases/owns the domain?	You should be the only one to purchase the domain. It's a red flag if the vendor offers to do this for you.
2. Who owns the content?	Again, the answer must be <u>you</u>. Except for stock images that the vendor may suggest licensing, you should own all content on the site. And this must clear in a written contract with the developer.
3. How do you ensure that all of our content and images are stored and transferred securely as you develop and maintain the site, and move content between servers?	The vendor should obtain SSL certificates for each connection between all of the platforms and systems they use for your site. A certificate validates that the connection points are secure and encrypted.
4. Which connections do you recommend be secured by SSL certificates?	This strengthens the answer to the previous question and the answer should be "all of them." Every server-to-Internet connection point should be secure and encrypted. That means anytime content or images are moved from your practice computers to the vendor's, or the vendor's to your website hosting company, all are secured by an SSL certificate.
5. Is the content management system (CMS) that you use encrypted and secure?	The answer should be yes.
6. Do you use Java or Adobe Flash?	The answer should be no to both. These are outdated technology tools and make a site easier to hack.
7. What do you know about encrypted email/messaging from the site's Contact Us form page? Which encryption services do you use for this kind of communication?	The vendor should demonstrate a basic understanding of how to encrypt the data transmitted from this form, as well as recommend using a Captcha on your Contact Us form.
8. What do you do to ensure security and HIPAA compliance within your company?	The vendor should demonstrate that they have done everything your practice has done to comply with HIPAA—because the HIPAA Omnibus Rule essentially requires all business associates to be a stringent as Covered Providers. Answers could include: require initial and annual HIPAA training for all employees and independent contractors; use secure, encrypted email when sending PHI; conduct an annual technical audit; developed a breach policy; or use strong passwords in all login credentials.
9. Describe the security of the website host you use.	The host should be willing to sign a BAA and provide evidence of HIPAA compliance. At a minimum, the hosting servers must store your data in a secure, encrypted environment.
10. Tell me what you do to ensure accessibility? Which guidelines do you follow?	The vendor should know about the WC3 guidelines for web accessibility. They should know about how visually and hearing-impaired people use devices to "read" the site. Answers about the "how" include: add contextual text to all images, offer multiple font sizes, and create clear content headers on all pages so devices can easily read them.
11. Where do you get the images used on the site? Is there an additional license fee for these?	There are many stock image sites. Some are free, but most require that the user pay a licensing fee. The developer should maintain a log of the images you've licensed or purchased and be able to produce it when requested.

Ask These Questions	Hope to Hear These Answers
12. Where and how often is the site backed up?	It should be backed up at least weekly and stored on a secure and encrypted server.
13. If we need to restore from a backup, how is this done? Tell me how the data stays secure.	The answer should include the process for uploading your data via a secure connection.
14. If we decide to part ways, in what format do you deliver all of our content and images, and what is the process for doing so?	The answer should include the process for uploading your data via a secure connection.

Liability.com Checklist

The checklist below is a homework assignment for all practices and their web developers:

1. Review and confirm that your site follows all of the security features recommended in this chapter, and that your web developer understands HIPAA compliance.
2. Verify that all communication channels—including all website forms—are encrypted and SSL certificates have been purchased for each connection.
3. Verify that all of your data is stored on a secure, encrypted server, and that it is backed up at least weekly.
4. Confirm you own the copyright or have licensed legal rights to all images appearing on your website. If you do not have the rights to an image, get the rights or remove the image. *No exceptions.*
5. Make sure your website has proper disclosures and that you've obtained consents from patients when required. You may want to add "Terms of Use." Your professional association may have templates to get you started.
6. If you haven't recently reviewed the BAA originally signed by the web developer, do so and make sure it follows the most recent HIPAA requirements. If you've never had a BAA with the web developer, get one signed as soon as possible.
7. Train your staff to be diligent about social engineering scams.
8. Audit your website for its compliance with accessibility guidelines. Start by using one of the many free or low-cost automated tools to check your site. The W3C has a list of these at: https://www.w3.org/WAI/ER/tools. Then, ask your web developer to arrange for a human review, either by someone with a disability or who has accessibility testing skills. Based on your findings, develop a plan for moving toward accessibility compliance. Address the "easy things" first and move toward full compliance as soon as you are able.

REFERENCES

1. Results of Google search conducted on February 21, 2018.
2. Staff. Largest healthcare data breaches of 2017. *HIPAA Journal*, January 4, 2018. https://www.hipaajournal.com/largest-healthcare-data-breaches-2017. Accessed May 6, 2018.
3. Leventhal R. Report: Healthcare accounted for 45% of all ransomware attacks in 2017. Healthcare Informatics website, https://www.healthcare-informatics.com/news-item/cybersecurity/report-health-care-accounted-45-all-ransomware-attacks-2017, Accessed February 22, 2018.
4. Wikipedia, "Social Engineering (security), https://en.wikipedia.org/wiki/Social_engineering_%28security %29. Accessed March 28, 2018.
5. These examples are from the Accessibility section of the W3C site page, Accessed March 29, 2018.

2. LICENSING BOARDS: ETHICAL DUTIES IN THE CYBER WORLD

∾

HIPAA Considerations and Best Practices to Avoid Breaches

CASE STUDIES: MISGUIDED MISTAKES AND EGREGIOUS ERRORS

When it comes to HIPAA violations, there are, sadly, plenty of examples available to serve as cautionary tales. Some seem like innocent mistakes that just about anyone could make. Others are so egregious that those involved appear to be willfully inviting the wrath of regulators and malpractice attorneys. Unfortunately, some people assume that any post that does not include the patient's name or photograph is a safe post. As we will see, that is a false and dangerous assumption. The following examples of HIPAA violations over the years offer valuable lessons for anyone dealing with patient privacy issues in the digital age.

Patient Privacy

The risks of venting on social media were made clear by an incident that took place nearly a decade ago. A shootout in Dearborn, Michigan, resulted in both a wounded police officer and a wounded suspect being rushed to Oakwood Hospital. The officer died, the suspect survived. After leaving work, Nurse Cheryl James logged onto Facebook and, in an emotional post, stated that she had come face-to-face with evil and hoped the (alleged) cop-killer would rot in hell.

James did not identify the hospital or the patient by name, nor did she reveal his medical condition. But the hospital administrators realized that, given the intense local press coverage of the event, the public could easily deduce both the patient's identity and where he was being treated. The nurse removed the post, but it was too little, too late. She was terminated for her actions. Remember, anytime someone can "connect the dots" in information you post and determine who a patient is, you are violating HIPAA.[1]

Hackers remain a growing, ever-present danger. There are plenty of hackers out there, but a group known as The Dark Overlord has become infamous for targeting medical entities. In 2016, its first year of existence, the group successfully attacked numerous healthcare providers in the U.S. and abroad. The next year, its victims included London Bridge Plastic Surgery, an exclusive UK practice with patients that include high-profile celebrities.

Dark Overlord hackers were able to access a photo database and steal photos of surgeries in progress, including breast and genitalia enhancements. The group claimed that members of the British Royal Family appeared in the stolen patient photos. Both the practice and police acknowledged the breach, and the practice apologized to its patients, but little information has emerged since. It is unclear if The Dark Overlord was paid off by the practice to withhold or return the material or if the hackers are simply biding their time, perhaps scheming to blackmail individual patients who appear in the photos.[2]

While I realize an event in the UK falls under British laws rather than HIPAA regulations, the patient privacy issues remain the same—and so do the precautions a provider must take. The best ways to defend against hackers are to back up systems daily, keep all software up-to-date, use strong password protection, encrypt data, ensure vendor compliance, and train your staff. To modify a line from Thomas Jefferson, the cost of patient privacy is eternal vigilance.

Before and After

Because purely cosmetic procedures are not typically covered by health insurance, plastic surgery practices often need to market their services more aggressively than other providers. This often means posting patient "before and after" photos in order to showcase a surgeon's results. Doing so can place the provider in the center of a digital minefield, where slip-ups can result in lawsuits and HIPAA violations.

Mandi Stillwell, a San Francisco photographer, was stunned when a man she met on an online dating site informed her that his Google search of her name had turned up photographs of her bare breasts. Stillwell had undergone plastic surgery in Fresno and had agreed in writing to let Dr. Enraquita Lopez photograph her and use the images to market the practice. However, the agreement stipulated that if images of her results were used, Stillwell would remain unidentifiable. The photographs showed only her torso.

Stillwell filed suit against Dr. Lopez. In court, Dr. Lopez's lawyer explained that the doctor and her staff had made a mistake and accidentally placed identifiable photos of Stillwell on the Internet. The photos were removed as soon as the doctor was made aware of them. The jury found in favor of Stillwell, and she was awarded an $18,000 settlement. Of course, just because the doctor had the photos removed from the Internet does not mean they will not reappear. Any viewer with a computer could have copied them and could repost them at any time.[3]

In 2013, Texas plastic surgeon Dr. James R. Motlagh performed liposuction on one of his employees. He photographed her prior to surgery, showing her face. He then shot video of her under anesthesia, capturing images of her naked torso. Prior to beginning the surgery, he posted this material on a professional association Facebook page. During the surgery, the hospital management was alerted to the post, and requested Dr. Motlagh immediately remove the images, but he was tied up performing the operation and could not.

The patient quit working for the practice and filed a lawsuit, claiming negligence and breach of privacy. Ironically, she was in charge of getting patients to sign off on forms allowing the use of their images for marketing. She had never signed such a form herself, though Dr. Motlagh apparently assumed she had. Both agreed that she had given Motlagh oral permission to photograph aspects of the surgery, but the patient claimed the conversation had made it clear that neither her identity nor her naked torso would be revealed. A jury awarded the patient $140,000+ in damages, and Dr. Motlagh was disciplined by the Texas Board of Medical Examiners.[4]

Even when a provider is confident that photos it has posted make it impossible to identify a patient, the digital world can prove them wrong. In one case, otherwise anonymous photos were posted on a practice's website in such a way that clicking on the photos revealed their digital file names, which included the patients' names. You must be aware of hidden or semi-hidden information in digital photos and other files and always make sure that all patient identifiers are removed.

An Inside Job

An employee who unintentionally creates a HIPAA breach is bad enough, but a rogue employee who willfully creates them is every practice's worst nightmare. Some employees can't resist snooping in medical records; others go much further.

Consider the case of a high-end plastic surgery practice located on Beverly Hill's posh Rodeo Drive. A contract employee who started out as a driver and translator was soon given other duties, including data entry. Things went bad very quickly.

Just six months after the employee started, the practice confronted her about missing funds. She quit but claimed she could not return her company phone because she had lost it. The practice was able to recover the phone when the ex-employee was caught trespassing at a facility that stored patient records. According to the office manager, the former employee had been surreptitiously photographing and videoing patients and procedures, patient records, and credit card numbers. It also appears the employee may have been responsible for a burglary at the practice, during which a large amount of data was downloaded to a hard drive and paper records were stolen. Some patients began receiving threatening and harassing phone calls and emails. As of this writing, the Los Angeles Sheriff's Department is conducting an ongoing investigation.[5,6]

Obviously, you should screen and background check employees carefully to help prevent "inside jobs." And every employee should be thoroughly trained and know the boundaries that apply to their position. What's more, you should be monitoring data access to ensure that no one is viewing, printing, or downloading any information that is beyond the scope of their duties. Doing so allows you to spot irregularities early on and deal with them in a timely manner.

24/7 Connections

When cellphones first became widely affordable, American popular culture coined the phrase "don't drink and dial," warning those who suddenly had 24/7 mobile phone access that a spur-of-the-moment call to express love or disdain for an ex, a boss, a co-worker, or a casual acquaintance is a very bad idea. Today, the cellphone is a smartphone with a digital camera, texting, and access to the Internet, including email and social media platforms. With that kind of instantaneous communications power in everybody's pocket, everywhere they go, it's no surprise that numerous HIPAA violations are smartphone-related. In certain circumstances, even the most buttoned-down employee can fall victim to the temptation of inappropriate, instantaneous communication. Every healthcare provider should have a firm policy in place regarding the carrying and use of personal phones in the workplace.

In December 2016, a patient underwent surgery at the University of Pittsburgh Medical Center's Bedford Memorial Hospital to remedy a strange injury—an object had been inserted into his penis, and part of the object was protruding from the organ. During the surgery, a doctor requested a photo of the injury be taken with the operating room camera for teaching purposes. He was told the camera was not working, and a number of operating room staffers began photographing the injury with their cellphone cameras. It appears that some of these individuals were in the OR to view the novel injury rather than out of medical necessity. Others were attempting to get a gander from outside the OR doors.

The photos were soon being sent to other hospital staffers' phones. One employee finally got fed up and reported the photo-sharing to management. The story broke in the press and spread quickly. The hospital investigated and self-reported the HIPAA violation. Employees were disciplined and the surgical services nursing director was replaced. Ironically, the investigation found that the OR camera was not out of order; it was so difficult to use that the staff had assumed it was broken.[7,8]

Questionable Judgment

What may well be the most egregious example of a HIPAA violation in recent memory comes not from a private practice or local hospital, but from the U.S. armed forces. In September of 2017, two white female junior enlisted corpsmen at the Jacksonville Naval Hospital in Jacksonville, Florida, were taking care of newborns in the nursery. Incredibly, they decided to use their smartphone cameras to amuse themselves at the infants' expense. One corpsman lifted an African American infant and manipulated the baby's arms to make it appear as if the child were dancing to a rap song playing on a cellphone while the other videoed the prank. One also took a picture of herself giving the infant "the finger." As if that weren't bad enough, the corpsmen then posted the material on social media, complete with captions referring to the infants under their care as "mini-satans."[9]

The women had uploaded their ugly stunt to Snapchat, a photo and video platform beloved by Millennials and Generation Z. Access to Snapchat posts can be limited to a specific audience, and the posts automatically disappear after a limited time. Apparently, the young women were confident that this would prevent their behavior from being viewed by anyone outside a small circle of select friends. They were wrong. A former school classmate saw the images and, angered by the mistreatment of newborns, was able to capture the material and post it on Facebook. The images went viral and were quickly seen by hundreds of thousands of people online.

The story made national and international news, and the images—with the infant's face now digitally obscured—appeared in print and online in major news publications. Appropriately appalled, the navy brass reacted quickly. The hospital's commanding officer removed the women from their duties, issued a public apology, and notified the parents of the infant whose image was posted. Vice Admiral Forrest Faison, the navy's surgeon general, ordered a 48-hour stand down of all Navy Medicine's commands to "review our oaths, our pledges, our reasons for serving, as well as Navy Medicine's policy regarding use of personally owned phones and other recording devices." He made it clear that the perpetrators would be prosecuted, most likely under both the codes of military and civilian justice, and he banned the presence of all workers' personal phones in patient areas.[10]

Bond of Trust

The lessons of this notorious incident and the others I've covered are crystal clear. You must be absolutely sure that you, your partners, and your employees all understand that both the practice of medicine and patient privacy laws are serious business. Patients literally trust you and your staff with their health and their lives; they should certainly be able to trust you with their privacy. A patient's personal health information is not grist for self-promotion, humor, or personal or political opinions, online or anywhere else. HIPAA compliance not only protects patient privacy, it protects the bond of trust between you and your patients.

FIGURE III-4. On Guard Online: Cybersecurity Basics

1. **Take Passwords Very Seriously**—Failing to use passwords, or using weak passwords, is more than an open invitation to digital intruders, it is failure to meet HIPAA's current standard of care.
2. **Train Your Employees**—Make your employees understand the importance of patient privacy and train them to use all equipment, systems, and communications properly in order to protect that privacy.
3. **Back Up Your Systems**—Backing up your systems regularly ensures your ability to restore information if it is seized by hackers using the malware known as "ransomware." Regular back-ups also prevent loss of information due to accidents such as computer crashes.
4. **Keep All Software Up-to-Date**—Routine software updates often include "patches" that fix security vulnerabilities. Make sure that every software update is installed as soon as possible.
5. **Encrypt Information and Communications**—Encryption is essential, especially when medical information appears on a mobile device or on a USB drive or any form of external hard drive. If you choose to communicate with or about a patient via text or email, you must use HIPPA-approved, encrypted formats and should have a patient's written permission to do so.
6. **Know Your Mobile**—Mobile devices should be secured under lock and key when not in use. Keep a list of all device serial numbers and who has access to them and a "checkout" log for shared devices. Many mobile devices include a tracking feature that can be used locate them if they go missing. Make sure the tracking feature is turned on when devices are set up for use. Finally, make sure devices are set up for remote erasure should timely recovery prove impossible.
7. **Use USB Drives with Care**—Any information on a USB or any other form of external drive absolutely must be encrypted. All computers and devices should be set up to scan any drive for viruses and malware before accessing the information on the drive. Any "auto-play" feature on a computer or device that triggers immediate play should always be turned off.
8. **Consider a File Sharing System**—A file sharing system allows your practice to eliminate the use of external drives, including USB drives. It also lets you know who is accessing material and when.

9. **Beware of Hidden Hard Drives**—Hard drives are everywhere—in security cameras, answering machines, scanners, copiers, medical devices, and more. Any of these hard drives may be recording electronic protected health information (ePHI), with or without you realizing it. They can also offer hackers a "back door" into your systems. Identify all hard drives associated with your practice and make sure they are password protected whenever possible and disposed of properly when no longer in use.

10. **Beware of Free Wi-Fi in Public Places**—Public Wi-Fi networks in Starbucks, Dunkin' Donuts, and other national chains, as well as hotels, libraries, and airports, may not be secure, and can put ePHI at risk. Always turn off any computer or mobile device feature that automatically searches for and connects with Wi-Fi networks.

11. **Use Only HIPAA-Compliant Vendors**—Any vendor you use must understand the ramifications of HIPPA and sign a HIPAA agreement with your practice.

12. **Make a Plan and Appoint a Cyber-Crisis Manager**—Cyber breaches arrive unexpectedly and dealing with them is time consuming and expensive. You should have a response plan in place before one occurs. You should also appoint and train an individual who will take charge of notifying the authorities and remedying the situation if you suffer a hack, HIPAA violation, or other cyber crisis. Make sure your cyber-crisis manager has the authority and resources he or she needs to succeed.

13. **Purchase Robust Cyber Insurance from a Qualified Vendor**—A business cyber insurance policy that covers online breaches will not only help with costs, it will put you in touch with experts who have dealt with breaches before. Avoid cyber policies that sound too good to be true. They may be inexpensive, but that's because they deliver little protection.

14. **Conduct a HIPAA Risk Assessment Annually**—Your HIPAA risk assessment is one of the first things the Office of Civil Rights will request should they ever come knocking. Woe to the practice that does not have one to show them.

REFERENCES

1. Katarsky, C. Nurse fired for HIPPA violation after discussing cop-killer patient: Was it fair? *Healthcare Business News*, August 24, 2010. http://www.healthcarebusinesstech.com/nurse-fired-for-hipaa-violation-after-discussing-cop-killer-patient. Accessed May 6, 2018.

2. Cox, J. Hackers steal photos from plastic surgeon to the stars, claim trove includes royals. *The Daily Beast*, October 23, 2017. https://www.thedailybeast.com/hackers-steal-photos-from-plastic-surgeon-to-the-stars-claim-they-include-royals. Accessed May 6, 2018.

3. Lopez, P. What's the penalty for posting a woman's breasts on Google? Just $18,000. *The Fresno Bee*, August 14, 2017. https://www.fresnobee.com/news/local/article165969457.html. Accessed February 14, 2018.

4. Staff. Tyler patient awarded $140,000, plastic surgeon posts video of her in operating room on Facebook. *KYTX/Tyler Morning Telegraph*, May 25, 2017. http://www.cbs19.tv/article/news/local/tyler-patient-awarded-140000-plastic-surgeon-posts-video-of-her-in-operating-room-on-facebook/442984310. Accessed May 6, 2018.

5. Wick, J. Massive security breach at Rodeo Drive plastic surgery clinic puts thousands of patient files at risk. *LAist*, June 1, 2017. http://laist.com/2017/06/01/clinic_breach.php. Accessed May 6, 2018.

6. Johnson. S. Beverly Hills plastic surgery clinic rocked by patient records heist: 'There is still outstanding stolen property.' *Hollywood Reporter*, June 8, 2017. https://www.hollywoodreporter.com/news/beverly-hills-plastic-surgery-identity-theft-is-still-outstanding-stolen-material-1011301. Accessed May 6, 2018.

7. Staff. Hospital staff circulated photos of patient's genital injury, investigation reveals. *Fox News*, September 14, 2017. http://www.foxnews.com/health/2017/09/14/hospital-staff-circulated-photos-patients-genital-injury-investigation-reveals.html. Accessed May 6, 2018.

8. Staff. Hospital staff discovered to have taken and shared photographs of patient's genital injury. *HIPAA Journal*, September 15, 2017. https://www.hipaajournal.com/hospital-staff-discovered-taken-shared-photographs-patients-genital-injury-8968. Accessed May 6, 2018.

9. Magness, J. 'Mini-Satans': Why is this 'Navy nurse' giving a newborn baby the middle finger? *The Miami Herald*, September 19, 2017. http://www.miamiherald.com/news/nation-world/national/article174085371.html. Accessed May 6, 2018.

10. Finley, T. Navy hospital removes staffers for calling babies mini-satans on social media. *The Huffington Post*, September 20, 2017. https://www.huffingtonpost.com/entry/hospital-staff-post-images-of-black-newborns-dancing-to-rap-refer-to-them-as-satans_us_59c2cfede4b06f93538c2c03. Accessed May 6, 2018.

∼

Overview of the Federation of State Medical Boards' *Model Guidelines for the Appropriate Use of Social Media and Social Networking in Medical Practice*

In April of 2012, the Federation of State Medical Boards adopted a new policy and issued a corresponding report. *Model Guidelines for the Appropriate Use of Social Media and Social Networking in Medical Practice* is the organization's codification of a commonsense approach to the use of social media and networking by physicians and healthcare professionals.

Professional ethics and etiquette form the core of the *Model Guidelines for the Appropriate Use of Social Media and Social Networking in Medical Practice*. Despite the lengthy official title, the guidelines are refreshingly brief, straightforward, and succinct. They offer a firm foundation on which to build the specifics of your practice's social media policy. Following them demonstrates your willingness to adhere to "industry standards" for cybersecurity, online behavior, and patient privacy.

For reference, the *Model Guidelines for the Appropriate Use of Social Media and Social Networking in Medical Practice* appear in full in this book. You and your staff would be wise to review them, adopt them as policy, and cover them in your employee training. This overview is provided to introduce the guidelines and summarize the policies detailed within them. It should not be a substitute for familiarizing yourself with the full policy document.

ISSUES AND ANSWERS

The *Model Guidelines* were created to allow medical professionals to make the most of the opportunities that social media and networking create. They do so by defining boundaries and eliminating grey areas that can damage the doctor-patient relationship or result in privacy breaches. The *Model Guidelines* also address other online issues and behaviors that can damage a practice's reputation.

According to results stated in the *Model Guidelines*, a 2010 survey found that 92% of state medical boards had dealt with reported violations of online professionalism. The most common violations were:

- Use of Internet for inappropriate contact with patients;
- Inappropriate prescribing;
- Misrepresentation of credentials; and
- Misrepresentation of clinical outcomes.

Responses to these violations by the individual state medical boards ranged from informal warnings to formal disciplinary proceedings. The disciplinary proceedings were serious matters, some of which resulted in license limitations, suspension, or revocation.

Areas that the document cites as needing to be addressed include:

- Protecting patient privacy and confidentiality (HIPAA);
- Avoiding requests for online medical advice;
- Acting professionally;
- Being upfront and accurate regarding employment, credentials, and conflicts of interest; and
- Being aware that online material may be available to anyone and can be misconstrued.

BASIC GUIDELINES

The *Model Guidelines* address doctor-patient relationships first, noting that in the digital era, such a relationship may begin online rather than in person. This means that both the doctor and the patient must be able to firmly establish their respective identities when communicating electronically. Of equal importance, physicians must be aware that standards of medical care *do not change* based upon the means of doctor-patient communication.

Physicians must always be aware that even online interactions that appear innocuous or trivial may violate the doctor-patient relationship. Remember, medical professionals should never use their position to develop personal relationships with patients—online or off. Nor should they ever portray themselves in an unprofessional light.

What *should* physicians do online? The *Model Guidelines* refer back to the Federation of State Medical Boards' previously issued guidelines for medical websites:

- **Be Candid:** Clearly disclose any financial, personal, or professional information that could influence a patient's understanding or use of information gained from your website or social media accounts.
- **Respect Privacy:** Do everything in your power to protect patient and personal data. Make sure that "de-identified" data cannot be traced back to a patient or user. Also, remember that a patient's online disclosure of his or her health information does not grant the practice the right to make additional disclosures.
- **Maintain Integrity:** Never place misleading, confusing or deceptive material online. Keep content clear, concise, and up-to-date. Indicate whether information is based on studies, consensus, professional experience, or personal opinion.

DOCTORS AND PATIENTS ONLINE

What about physician-patient interaction online? The *Model Guidelines* discourage any interaction with current or past patients on personal social networking platforms, such as Facebook, Instagram, and Twitter. They strongly recommend restricting any online contact with patients to accepted forms of online professional communication regarding treatment.

Have a quick discussion about social media and patient privacy with all new and existing patients. Be brief, but make it clear that professional ethics prevent you from engaging in activities such as "friending" them on Facebook, viewing their family vacation photos on Instagram, commenting on their tweets etc. Be sure patients understand that this is not a personal judgment about them, and that you're actually following both a code of conduct and solid legal advice in order to protect their privacy and medical confidentiality.

Remember that patients are people, and people are social animals. Nearly all of us seek friendship and want to be well liked and well thought of. Doctors and patients bond in unique ways—particularly when dealing with serious or long-term illnesses and conditions. It's easy to understand how telling a patient you can't be their Facebook friend could lead to anger or hurt feelings on their part, so don't forget your bedside manner when addressing this issue. Be polite but firm. You may even want to blame your medical board. "I would like to connect directly on Facebook, but I can't. Believe or not, the state licensing board prohibits doctors becoming Facebook friends with patients. I'm sorry."

MEDICAL DISCUSSIONS

When it comes to discussing medicine online, the *Model Guidelines* are bracingly firm: Never do so on personal social media! Stick to professional online platforms, such as Doximity. This professional platform for physicians allows you to exchange HIPAA-compliant messages and images and discuss the latest treatment guidelines and medical news.

Just remember, you are responsible for reviewing any professional site's protections, complying with its terms of use, and creating effective password protection when accessing such a site. You are also responsible for confirming the validity of any medical information from such a site before incorporating it into your practice. If you currently use Facebook Messenger to answer a patient's medical question, you fail.

PATIENT PRIVACY

The *Model Guidelines* clearly state that you should never use social media in any way that could lead to patient identification. Online breaches of patient privacy via social media can expose protected information to a massive audience in a very short time. The *Model Guidelines* reiterate that, if you think referring to a patient by using a code name, nickname, or room number will prevent that individual from being identified, you are wrong. They also state that posting a patient's photo is an invitation to disaster.

FULL DISCLOSURE

The *Model Guidelines* also cover disclosure. Should you choose to write about your experiences in healthcare, online or in print, you must reveal any conflicts of interest. You must also state your professional credentials clearly and accurately.

POSTING CONTENT

When posting content, you must be aware that it may be widely disseminated and could "live" in the digital world forever. That's a sobering thought, since anything you post is also subject to misunderstanding, misinterpretation, and being taken out of context. This is why you must always avoid posting inaccurate, outdated, or ambiguous information.

The security, privacy and confidentiality of the material is your responsibility as well. Your professionalism is tantamount, both as a healthcare professional and an author. If you are creating content for an employer or online publication, you must familiarize yourself with their rights regarding reviewing, editing, posting, and deleting material. Should you choose to moderate a website, you must stay on top of it, properly policing and correcting comments on a regular basis.

PROFESSIONAL BEHAVIOR

The final section of the *Model Guidelines* deals with professional behavior. The key takeaway here is to separate your personal online presence and your professional online presence. Keep material on personal sites personal and professional sites professional. Make sure they are always separate and unique. The same goes for email. Use professional email addresses for professional communication and personal email addresses for personal communication. Do not allow the two to overlap—no mixing and matching!

At this point in the digital age, the other professional rules in the *Model Guidelines* should be no-brainers, but I'll repeat them just in case…

Act online as you would offline. No offensive, demeaning, sexist, or racist jokes, opinions, or language. No verbal attacks on patients or fellow medical professionals. No trolling, cyber-stalking, or cyber-bullying. No angry, bitter, or drunken venting. No presentation of, or praise for, irresponsible or illegal behavior. No bending or breaking of the stated policies of your state medical board, government regulators, insurance providers, hospitals, or other entities. In short, act like your mother will see everything you do online.

There is one more guideline that must be mentioned, though some physicians may balk at it. If you witness any unprofessional behavior by other medical professionals, you should report it to the proper authorities. In other words, no "code of silence."

Again, the complete *Model Guidelines for the Appropriate Use of Social Media and Social Networking in Medical Practice* appear in the index. Familiarizing yourself with them and following them are two of the smartest things you will ever do.

The complete Federation of State Medical Boards' Report is here: https://www.fsmb.org/globalassets/advocacy/policies/model-guidelines-for-the-appropriate-use-of-social-media-and-social-networking.pdf

3. PRACTICAL CYBERSECURITY FOR PHYSICIANS: HOW TO DEVELOP POLICIES, PROCEDURES, AND EFFECTIVE TRAINING

Are you certain that all staff members and physicians know how to recognize a phishing email? Is every mobile device, tablet, and laptop encrypted and password protected? Have you prepared your team to recognize and handle a social engineering scheme?

Based on my work with hundreds of physician practices, I'm guessing that you answered "no" to at least two of these questions. And I also understand the reasons why: The office is short staffed. The appointment schedule is overflowing. Perhaps your practice is small and lacks professional management.

But while just five years ago practices could take a calculated risk and "overlook" policy development or underfund employee training, cybercrime has hit a fever pitch these days. The prevalence of electronic health records (EHRs), cloud-based applications, and the Internet of Things (IoT) has increased the vulnerability of healthcare data. No matter if your practice is large or small, preparedness efforts such as developing policies and procedures and implementing ongoing employee training are essential to helping the practice avoid an attack that compromises your systems and results in stolen data or ransom demands.

This chapter focuses on the practical action steps that a hyper-busy physician or practice administrator can take to plug common preparedness gaps and develop the policies, procedures, and training necessary to maintain digital security measures. It addresses some of the most pressing questions I'm asked by practice leaders and physicians, including:

- Which are the highest-priority risks to focus on?
- What is an effective way to develop policies and procedures?
- What kind of training do we really need?
- Are annual generic HIPAA training modules enough or do we need to do more?
- How can we keep staff and physicians engaged and on high alert after training is over?

WHY PREPAREDNESS IS WORTH THE EFFORT

2017 was the "worst year ever" for cybersecurity incidents, according to the Online Trust Alliances' Cyber Incident & Breach Trends Report. Based on the number of reported breaches, the organization estimates that the number of cyber incidents was nearly double the number in 2016.[1] Further, the Identity Theft Resource Center recorded a total of 1,579 U.S. breaches in 2017—23.7% of which were in healthcare.[2]

Sadly, most healthcare organizations are woefully unprepared to deal with such cyber attacks. And according to leading cybersecurity expert James Scott, the most common weak spots in healthcare information security aren't due to a dearth of technical security features or tools. They stem from the practical, operational steps that must be taken on the front-line level of a practice or healthcare organization. The three most common weak spots are:

1. Lack of written policies and procedures.
2. Insufficient, relevant workforce training.
3. Lack of a thorough and timely risk analysis.[3]

According to the Ponemon Institute's *2017 Cost of a Data Breach Survey,* the average cost for each lost or stolen record containing sensitive and confidential information, across all industries, is $141 per record. However, the average cost per record in a *healthcare* organization is $380.[4] And that's in addition to potential HIPAA fines of $1.5M per incidence as well as the class action suits that could occur if the HIPAA violations involve more than 500 patient records. And finally, don't forget the cost and damage to your reputation. Studies indicate that the reputational hit from a data breach can cost you patients.

As the saying goes, an ounce of prevention is worth a pound of cure. Your practice can reduce the financial pain of a security breach by conducting an annual risk assessment, developing policies and procedures, training all staff and physicians, and implementing ongoing compliance checks and education. In fact, the Online Trust Alliances report claims that 93% of all U.S. data breaches last year could have been avoided with proper preparedness and due diligence.

This means preparing the practice and employees to identify, avoid, and take action when they recognize cyber issues such as phishing, social engineering attacks, and ransomware schemes. It also means assessing whether business associates have appropriate policies and procedures in place to protect your data. Remember, the HIPAA Omnibus Rule holds physicians accountable for ensuring that the business associates they contract with have appropriate privacy, security, and breach protocols in place.

FOCUS ON THE BIGGEST RISKS FIRST

If your practice has limited time and resources for preparedness, it might as well adopt the Willie Sutton approach to preparedness. Sutton was a successful bank robber in the early 1920s, making off with an estimated $2M in dough. When he was finally caught by the authorities, they asked him, "Willie, why did you rob all those banks?" To which Sutton reportedly replied: "Because that's where the money is."

This same targeted approach can work for practices that are developing preparedness material and training on a shoestring. *Focus on the biggest risk areas first.* Here are the top three:

Phishing

Data from *Verizon's 2017 Data Breach Investigations Report* indicates that 43% of all breaches (healthcare and other industries combined) are the result of a phishing scam.[5] By addressing just this one cyber threat, you'll decrease your cyber risk significantly.

Phishing scams are a type of email or social engineering attack whereby cyber attackers attempt to coerce people to release or send personal information, often by asking them to click on a link in an email or enter information into a website field/form. Information that phishing schemes attempt to gather includes a person's User ID and password, credit card number, address, and phone number.

When employees don't recognize the email as a scam and provide the requested data, cyber criminals have the keys to all kinds of kingdoms. Imagine for a moment how powerful your employee's login credentials would be to a criminal who could use them to remotely log into your practice or hospital network and access data and systems. The amount of damage that can be done quickly is significant.

But if employees are properly trained and on guard, they will be able to detect the majority of phishing scam emails before anything nefarious occurs. In many cases, the signs of a phishing scam are fairly easy to spot: misspellings, unusual grammatical structure, or domain names or file extensions that don't match.

Phishing scams have become more and more sophisticated, however, and attackers are make their emails and websites look more legitimate. They may have incorporated official logos or marketing phrases to make your employees think it is authentic. Despite the increased sophistication, there are multiple ways to focus your team's attention on identifying suspicious emails. We'll cover them later in this chapter.

Malicious Email Attachments

Some emails arrive into your network with a secret toy surprise attached: a nasty file packed with malicious software ("malware") that's designed to install itself once opened and wreak havoc on your network and systems.

An example is an email masquerading as a notice of nonpayment from a legitimate company or organization, perhaps even one that your employee uses, such as Netflix.com or Citibank. The subject line and email are written to provoke concern that a "payment is overdue" or that "services may be terminated" if the employee does not send payment immediately. Caught up in the emotion of thinking, "but I already paid that bill…" the employee opens the attachment and pure cyber evil ensues.

The Verizon report indicates that 66% of the malware linked to data breaches or other incidents (i.e., ransomware) was installed via malicious email attachments.[6] In other words, *more than half (51%) of breaches involved the installation and use of malicious software.* How do you kill a snake? Cut off its head. Focus on reducing the number of malicious email attachments opened and you will reduce the number of malware installations—which in turn will reduce the opportunity for breaches.

Device Theft

Mobile devices, laptops, and tablets can easily go missing, and device theft is a common way to steal patient data. The fact that nearly 99% of devices used by healthcare professionals lack any security protection[7] makes them veritable goldmines in the hands of a hacker.

Installing encryption, security, and remote data-wiping features on all your practice's devices will make your data much harder to syphon from a stolen device. This single, straightforward action will take a huge bite out of the risk that the electronic patient and financial data will end up in the hands of criminals.

Now that you know some of the most common ways thieves can steal your data, focus on developing (or refreshing) policies and procedures related to plugging these security leaks.

DEVELOP/UPDATE POLICIES

The first step toward getting all physicians and practice leaders on the same page about security and privacy issues is to develop a set of essential cybersecurity policies.

I am fully aware of the malaise that sets in when I suggest this to physicians. Policy development is not the most riveting activity. Yet, it is essential and here's why: Policies drive the development of procedures. Procedures are what training is based on. And, you can't train people on policies and procedures that you don't have.

Policies create a written expression of what physicians and practice leaders have agreed to. This "guidance from on high" essentially codifies agreed-upon rules and provides a unified, sanctioned message for staff to follow.

There are three primary policies to be concerned with relative to cybersecurity:

- Security policy (required under HIPAA)
- Social media policy
- Mobile device policy

There is no need to reinvent the wheel to create these policies. Templates have been included in Section V to get you started. The templates are intended to speed development and implementation. Review and discuss them *thoughtfully and thoroughly* and then customize them to your specific circumstances, taking into consideration the discussion points that follow.

SECURITY POLICY

This policy, required by HIPAA, should include the following content. Each item listed includes "best practice" recommendations for you to integrate into your customized security policy.

1. *Risk Analysis.* Engage a professional to conduct this analysis every year; resist the temptation to conduct it on your own. (Figure III-5 explains why I advise against DIY risk assessments.) Provide a written report to the practice Compliance Officer, who can take action on identified risks.

2. *Information System Activity Review.* Conduct a regular review of who has access to which information systems in the practice and why. Remove access or permission levels for staff who have access to more electronic records containing protected health information (ePHI) than they need to complete their tasks, who no longer need that access, or who have left the practice. Software analytics tools such as Maize Analytics

can make this easier by analyzing each user's access to your ePHI and alerting the practice to patterns that indicate a potential security risk.

3. *Workforce Security.* This policy clause should include multiple components, such as:
   - Make sure a manager or physician approves staff access to systems that include PHI.
   - Conduct background checks prior to hire to identify whether prospective employees have been engaged in criminal activity.
   - Limit access to PHI based on an employee's job responsibilities.
   - Terminate access to all systems and the facility when an employee leaves. This is often overlooked in busy practices. Make sure you disable **all** credentials on **all** information systems.

4. *Password Management.* Insist on strong passwords and change them regularly. Your policy should disallow staff to write passwords on Post-It Notes and stick them to the computer or desk or keep them handy in a desk drawer where they can be found easily.

5. *Business Associate Agreements (BAAs).* Make sure your BAA language is current, you have agreements with all vendors and third parties that have access to PHI, and that these business associates have appropriate measures in place to minimize theft and breach.

6. *System Updates.* Make it a policy to ensure all operating systems, browsers, and software versions are current and automatically search for and download anti-virus updates and patches. Do not allow use of out-of-date/unsupported operating systems and applications—they create a ripe opportunity for hackers to get in. Once software is no longer being supported by a manufacturer, criminals can exploit the old code, which will no longer be patched.

7. *Security Incident Procedures and Contingency Plan.* Develop and maintain both of these, which include detail about (among other things) restoring system backups, validating security incidents, and conducting root cause analysis of how an incident occurred.

FIGURE III-5. Just Say No to DIY Risk Assessments

You may think you are "saving money" by downloading a checklist and foregoing the expense of engaging an IT professional to conduct an assessment. But this is a mistake that could end up costing the practice a bundle.

Just as an internist is not trained to perform shoulder arthroscopy, practice administrators and physicians are not trained to conduct an IT risk assessment. Simply following a checklist is not sufficient because you "don't know what you don't know" about the items on the list. You run the risk of misinterpreting an assessment criterion or overlooking any prerequisites necessary to deem an item as "satisfactory."

Hiring a professional is worth the expense. If you don't already engage an IT consultant, most healthcare attorneys can provide a referral.

SOCIAL MEDIA POLICY

I receive more questions and requests concerning social media policies than any other privacy policy. It's essential from both a security and human resources management perspective that you clarify your policies with employees upon hire and provide ongoing reminders.

The "meat" of the social media policy is the *Online Professional and Personal Behavior Clause.* Based on my experience, the following are "best practice" recommendations for you to integrate:

1. Restrict employees from posting PHI on any social media channel. (Yes, it's stating the obvious, but still important to have in writing.)
2. Do not allow employees to provide medical advice or commentary of any kind, as themselves or by impersonating anyone in the practice (such as providing information "as if" they were the physician).
3. Prohibit employees from transmitting any material that they or your practice do not have a right to make available by law. Remember in July 2015 when NFL standout Jason Pierre Paul's medical records got released via Twitter while he was hospitalized in Florida? This is the type of behavior the policy should address.
4. Prohibit employees from endorsing any product or service or taking political or lobbying action that would in any way reference or implicate your practice.

Violation of the social media policy should be taken seriously and is grounds for dismissal. That should also be stated in the policy (this language is included in the template).

MOBILE DEVICE POLICY

A mobile device policy is often missing in physician practices. Given the number of smartphones, tablets, laptops, and other devices used by physicians, other clinicians, and staff, this policy is extremely important. Outlined below are the "best practice" recommendations to include.

1. *Security Requirement.* All employees who use a mobile device to conduct the duties of their job—whether the device is personal or practice-owned—are responsible for protecting sensitive data from being lost or stolen. Employees are required to:
   - Install a password on all devices.
   - Configure a timeout of no more than 30 seconds.
   - Install remote location and wiping features on all devices. If the device is misplaced or stolen, these tools allow it to be found and/or the data to be remotely deleted— hopefully before a criminal gets access to it.
   - Encrypt the device whenever possible. Kaspersky Lab (kaspersky.com) is an option for PC, Mac, and Android devices.
   - Ensure the device data are being backed up regularly and that the backup system is working and HIPAA compliant.
   - Install anti-virus software on the device whenever possible. Norton Mobile Security (norton.com) and Kaspersky Lab are two options.

2. *Prohibited Uses.* Although certainly these functions are useful, in the healthcare workplace, it's wise to prohibit employees from using the camera, texting, and storing patient data on their mobile device. You could consider offering a secure message system as an alternative to the native texting apps on mobile devices. More and more EHR vendors offer these options, as do physician-patient engagement and communication apps such as HealthLoop, PatientPing, TigerConnect, or OhMD.

3. *Prohibited Locations.* To minimize distraction, your policy should list the areas where mobile devices are not allowed—for instance, in a room where a patient is undergoing an invasive procedure.

A framework for developing the Template Gallery policy templates into final documents is shown in Figure III-6. After you've customized (or refreshed) them, send the final version out for review by a healthcare attorney familiar with privacy and security laws in your state. After legal review, put them in a policy manual or incorporate them into an employee handbook—your choice. Less important than where you store them is how effectively you implement them by developing procedures and training.

Review and update the policies annually, based on changing federal regulations and the evolution of the practice.

FIGURE III-6. Policy Development Framework

1. **Choose a "document owner."** Typically, this is the practice administrator, but does not have to be. This individual's role is to integrate feedback into the template policies, distribute a version for review, integrate edits, and finalize the document after attorney review.

2. **Create a multi-disciplinary review team to provide input and edits.** Four to five individuals is about right. If your practice is small, two or three can work. The team should include representatives from physician leadership, IT (such as your IT consultant), staff, compliance officer, and administrator. A healthcare attorney does not need to be part of the team, but he or she will need to weigh in on questions and ultimately review the policies before you put them into place.

3. **Review the templates against your existing policies. Discuss issues, ask questions, define your specific issues/needs, and note them for inclusion in the policy.** Don't rush this process. It might take several review meetings, but a few hours spent hashing through the issues can save hundreds of hours and thousands of dollars cleaning up the mess after a data breach or phishing attack.

4. **Customize the template policies with your practice's specific circumstances; they should be unique to you and understood by all.** For many years, most practices implemented primarily generic policies that were put into a binder and sat on a shelf to collect dust. In today's climate of cyber crime, your practice must take policy development more seriously and rigorously customize the policies to your practice.

5. **Send the final version for attorney review.** Make sure the attorney you choose is familiar with privacy and security laws in your state.

Getting the policy part right will save you time creating procedures and training materials. Expect to go through several versions of this document before your attorney provides final feedback.

WRITTEN PROCEDURES ARE A MUST

Policies provide the "what" to do; procedures are the "how" do do it. Although policies and procedures are related, they are in fact two distinct sets of documents.

For example, if your policy is that *"employees must create strong passwords for network login,"* the procedure would describe how to set up a password that *"does not contain words from the dictionary or the employee's name and contains a minimum of eight characters that are a mix of upper and lowercase, numbers, and special symbols."*

In other words, procedures take the policy and translate it into instructions that indicate how something gets done. After policies have been approved, use them as the basis for developing procedures.

Here are two examples of high-priority procedures. Review them for their structure and clarity, and customize them for your practice. Use the structure of these policies to develop additional security policies for your organization.

FIGURE III-7. Sample Password Procedure

Using weak passwords threatens the privacy and security of our patient data. Weak passwords are easy for a hacker to "crack" and potentially breach our systems and databases. The following are common characteristics of weak passwords:

- Contain words found in the dictionary.
- Contain a word or number that is something personal to you: name, date, city, state.
- Contain common phrases.
- Do not contain enough character diversity (i.e., all lowercase).

Our practice policy is to create strong passwords with a minimum of eight characters. Here is how to do that:

- **Do not** use common words or phrases, dictionary words, or words such as your street name, child or pet's name, birthdate, or other information that could be easily guessed.
- **Do** use a combination of upper- and lowercase letters, at least one number, and at least one symbol.

In addition:

- **Do not** write down your password. Memorize it.
- **Do not** keep your password on a piece of paper in your desk drawer or on your desk.
- **NEVER** share your password with anyone.
- Our system will automatically remind you to update your password every quarter.

If you suspect your password may have been stolen, email or call our Director of Information Services, Jennifer Jaypeg, at 555-1212 immediately.

FIGURE III-8. Sample Procedure for Avoiding Phishing Scams

Phishing is a cyber threat that uses email to deceive people into disclosing passwords, bank account or credit card numbers, or other sensitive data. When a link within a phishing email is clicked, it may send you to a malicious website, or automatically begin a download of malware into our network.

To avoid the threat of phishing, be alert to emails that:

- Have subject lines that include words such as "Read This Now" or "Final Notice"
- Include poor grammar, misspelled words, overly formal greetings, or odd sentence construction.
- Contain attachments or links that have file extensions that don't match those of the sender, or "just don't look right."
- Appear to be from a government, bank, or other legitimate authority, but links or logos aren't official.
- Ask you to click on a link to update or validate information.
- Threaten you with dire consequences or offer a monetary reward.

If you receive an email with one or more of these suspicious characteristics, do not:

- Open the email or the attachment.
- Click on any links within the email.
- Call any telephone numbers in the email.
- Chare any of our practice's information, nor any of your own personal information.

If you suspect you have received a phishing or other suspicious email, ***do not forward the email.*** Call or create a new email to alert our IT Consultant, Ted Technology, at 555-1212 immediately.

DESIGN AN EFFECTIVE TRAINING PROGRAM

With policies and procedures marked as "done" on your to-do list, the next step toward preparedness is training physicians and staff. Keep in mind that to be effective, security training is different than training for other needs.

Most practices structure their cybersecurity training like they do other training—such as how to do CPR. Employees are given a comprehensive course, and provided annual refreshers or updates. But although CPR is "one and done" training (once you learn it, you know how to do it), **cybersecurity is just the opposite.** In order for employees to remember how to identify phishing, malicious attachments, and other scams, they must be reminded of the threat consistently.

Therefore, cybersecurity training is much more effective when it is delivered in *shorter sessions, more frequently, with ongoing reminders to keep employees on alert.*

So, although your training program does not need to be complex or fancy, it does need to be ongoing and multifaceted, and include basic training (online or live), quizzes, job aids, periodic scenario tests, and refresher training. It also must be customized to your practice's specific policies, procedures, and circumstances. **Offering generic HIPAA training alone is not enough.**

Developing this training material is not as complicated as you might think. You don't need beautiful, graphically elegant slides. The material can be as simple as a printed copy of your security, social media, and mobile device policies, your most essential procedures, and a short quiz at the end to test learning. A small practice might review this material one-on-one with new employees. If your practice is larger, perhaps you'll conduct a group training session.

Regardless of how you deliver the material, when combined with the generic, online HIPAA training that many practices purchase these days, you'll have a good set of foundational material for training new employees and delivering annual HIPAA refresher training to all employees.

Next, enhance this basic training by periodically distributing job training aids. Certainly your team will remember key training elements for a few days or weeks after completing the course. But two months and 898 emails later, they are busy caring for patients or appealing denied claims. Identifying a phishing email or possible ransomware attack is the last thing on their minds.

A job training aid like the one in Figure III-9 can be printed and put on employee desks, discussed in meetings, or used as a pop quiz. It will build employee knowledge through repetition, which is the key to security training success.

FIGURE III-9. Job Training Aid: How to Catch a Phish

The success of a phishing attack against our practice hinges on your ability to discern the difference between a legitimate and illegitimate information request in an email. Here are five of the most common elements of a phishing email. **If you notice them, do not click on any links or open any attachments. Contact our IT Administrator immediately.**

1. **Poor grammar and spelling.** If the email reads like a poor translation into English or has misspellings and odd grammar, it is likely a phishing email.
2. **A request for personal information.** Reputable companies do not ask for passwords, account numbers, or the answer to a security question. If the email contains any of these questions, it's probably malicious.
3. **Mismatched URLs.** If you hover your mouse over the top of the URL, you should see the actual hyperlinked address (at least in Outlook). If the hyperlinked address is different from the address that is displayed, the message is probably fraudulent or malicious.
4. **Domains that just aren't quite right.** If the email says it's from Wells Fargo Bank, but when you hover over links in the email you can see you are being directed to something other than the company's legitimate domain—like this: www.wellsfargo. johnsmaliciouswebsite.com—it's probably malicious. Don't click.
5. **Strange or unlikely senders.** For example, you receive an email from the CEO of a large company making a donation request. Or a government agency insisting that you follow some new law. If you didn't send an email message to either, it's probably a phish.

ONGOING TRAINING AND MONITORING ARE CRITICAL

How can you continuously keep security on the radar as a clear and present danger? Ongoing monitoring, regular reminders, and a discussion of breaches that have hit the national media are a few things that can be effective. The goal is to imprint in employees' minds that your practice takes cybersecurity very, very seriously—because the threat to your patients' privacy is very, very real.

By consistently reminding and re-training employees about the highest risks, you'll maintain awareness and reduce the threat of attacks. Here are a few practical ways to do this:

1. **Send periodic emails with reminders and tips.** Mark your calendar every six weeks with a reminder to send these out. Sending in the morning is most effective. For instance, remind employees not to write passwords on Post-It Notes and stick them to monitors. Or, send a 3-question quiz just prior to a staff meeting (the answers are presented in the meeting). You can easily pull reminders and tips from your policies and procedures.

2. **Conduct Phishing Tests.** These tests send emails to all employees in the network with fake phishing scams. Their purpose is to see how many people will click. The cybersecurity training company Knowbe4 (knowbe4.com) offers a free tool for this: Phishing Security Tool. They provide the file for your IT staff to transmit the fake phishing message and reporting that shows how many people clicked. Great for discussion in a staff meeting after the test is conducted.

3. **Administer periodic online tests to employees.** Again, Knowbe4 has a free tool: Automated Security Awareness Program (ASAP). Your IT staff or administrator uses their content and online tool to customize up to 25 questions.

4. **Print Posters and Reminders.** One practice I worked with created colorful "Watch Out for Phishing" posters and hung them on bathroom stall doors, in break rooms, and on bulletin boards.

5. **Have a "Catch the Phish" Award.** Award a $25–$50 gift certificate to each employee who spots—but does not click—a phishing scam. Announce the award in a staff meeting and discuss the issue as part of ongoing awareness.

6. **Put reminders in company communications.** If your practice sends a monthly newsletter to employees, include a story about security in several issues each year.

7. **Monitor employee password strength.** Knowbe4 has a free tool for this: Weak Password Test (WPT). WPT checks your Active Directory for several different types of weak password related threats, providing insight to the effectiveness of your password policies and any fails, so you can take action.

8. **Quarterly (Verbal) Cyber Awareness Quiz.** Make cyber hygiene fun by tossing out questions during quarterly staff meetings and asking the team for verbal answers. For example:
   a. "Name two common human error reasons that cyber attacks or breaches occur in healthcare."
   b. "What are two clues that an email may be a phishing email?"
   c. "What is ransomware and how does it work?"

Choosing just one or two of these ideas for ongoing monitoring will improve the retention of your training efforts and keep employees on alert for potential security threats.

CONCLUSION

Employees are a practice's weakest link in the effort to maintain cybersecurity. Reduce the risk by being prepared and maintaining awareness. Develop customized policies and procedures that reflect your practice's specific circumstances. Use the practical techniques from this chapter to create training material and job aids that go beyond generic HIPAA modules.

Most importantly, be sure to discuss security regularly and disseminate periodic reminders, tips, and scenario tests to keep employees on their toes. Doing so can keep cybersecurity at the top of every physician and staff person's mind—so they think twice about clicking.

REFERENCES

1. Staff. 2017 worst year ever for cybersecurity incidents according to online trust alliance. *HIPPA Journal*, February 1, 2018. https://www.hipaajournal.com/2017-worst-year-ever-cybersecurity-incidents-according-online-trust-alliance/. Accessed May 4, 2018

2. ITRC. *2017 annual data breach year-end review*. Identity Theft Resource Center. https://www.idtheftcenter.org/2017-data-breaches. Accessed May 4, 2018.

3. Although this chapter does not cover the topic of risk assessment, I strongly recommend that practices prioritize the completion of such an assessment annually. It's an essential component of a practice's security and privacy efforts and should be conducted with the support of an IT consultant or information security specialist.

4. Ponemon Institute. *2017 cost of data breach survey*. Ponemon Institute, June 2017. https://www-01.ibm.com/common/ssi/cgi-bin/ssialias?htmlfid=SEL03130WWEN&. Accessed May 4, 2018.

5. Verizon. *Verizon's 2017 data breach investigations report*. https://healthitsecurity.com/news/verizon-finds-phishing-attacks-malware-top-data-breach-causes. Accessed May 4, 2018.

6. Verizon's 2017 Data Breach Investigations Report

7. Scott, J. Cybersecurity hygiene for the healthcare industry. Self-Published, 2015, page 22.

Patient Satisfaction and Online Reviews—Managing Risk and Your Online Presence

One cannot underestimate the power of online reviews. How many of us would book a reservation at a new hotel or restaurant without consulting websites such as TripAdvisor or Open Table and reading what other people say about the places we are considering?

The same is true of our healthcare experiences and patients looking for a healthcare provider are no different than those customers looking for a restaurant or hotel. Studies have shown that a significant number of patients who are looking for a new provider want to know what current or former patients have to say. The growing popularity of online reviews is having a marked effect on how physicians practice.

A 2013 study by PriceWaterhouseCoopers indicates a heavy consumer reliance on online reviews as part of their decision-making process. Among 1,000 respondents, about half (48%) said they read healthcare reviews, and more than two-thirds of those—68%—said they used online reviews to help make healthcare decisions.[1] A German study showed that about 65% of patients surveyed said they had chosen a particular physician based on positive ratings.[2]

A recent survey conducted by Software Advice showed the 82% of patients use online reviews to evaluate physicians, and that 72% of patients use online reviews as the first step in finding a new doctor.[3]

Some of the more popular review websites patients use to express their opinions about the healthcare they received are Rate MDs, HealthGrades, Yelp, ZocDoc, Vitals, Angie's List, Dr. Score, Google Reviews, WebMD, and CareDash. Among the factors they rate are[2]:

- How the patient was treated by the medical staff;
- Patient wait time;
- Doctors attitude;
- The patient's level of trust in the doctor's decisions; and
- Patient's treatment results.

These detailed ratings have produced changes in the way physicians practice today. It is no longer sufficient to merely list the practice in the Yellow Pages or even have a good website. Studies have shown that customer service, and not clinical skill, provides the leading distinction between providers who are highly rated from those that are poorly rated. One study found that 96% of patient's complaints are related to customer service![2]

The growing use of online reviews has caused many healthcare providers to seek help from firms that offer online reputation management services and to make online reputation management a key part of their marketing budget. Although these firms use software to monitor online reviews, it is difficult to remove a negative review. Instead, best practices today call for healthcare providers to manage and improve their online reputation proactively. It's a great example of how an ounce of prevention is better than a pound of cure. (More tips on establishing your online reputation can be found later in this chapter.)

PATIENT SATISFACTION AS A VITAL METRIC

Hospitals and practices have conducted patient satisfaction surveys for years. Press Ganey is one well-known company that works with hospitals and physician groups to conduct these surveys. They perform formal surveys and produce case studies, webinars, and other resources designed to help medical practices improve patient satisfaction.

In recent years, patient satisfaction has gained increasing attention from executives across the healthcare industry and from the federal government. Hospitals began reporting their Hospital Consumer Assessment of Healthcare Providers and Systems (HCAHPS) scores 10 years ago and since fall 2012, Medicare has based its reimbursements in part on these measures. These new rules have raised the stakes for patient satisfaction surveys and caught increasing attention from executives across the healthcare industry.

Patient satisfaction as a measure of quality care is complex and controversial, and the debate will certainly continue and evolve as more data become available.

What is not debatable is the importance of providers' online reputation. Because of the emphasis on patient satisfaction as a measure of quality care, providers can no longer relegate it to periodic surveys or ignore it altogether. The growth of the online ratings business has made it easier for patients to describe their healthcare experiences in detail and to express their satisfaction—or lack of satisfaction.

In addition, patient satisfaction ratings have grown in importance because the metrics used are similar to those already used by the Center for Medicare and Medicaid Services (CMS) and sure to affect individual physicians in the future. Why not address these issues now?

Soliciting patient feedback, listening to patients talk about both the positive and negative experiences, and using those observations to improve your practice is a good way to improve patient satisfaction and safeguard your online reputation. A study of over 5,000 primary care patients a few years ago identified seven traits of physician excellence that directly affected patient satisfaction as reflected in their ratings of physicians: access, communication, personality and demeanor of provider, quality of medical care processes, care continuity, quality of healthcare facilities, and office staff.[4]

Empathy is another driver of positive physician ratings. A group at Massachusetts General Hospital studied the effectiveness of empathy training for resident physicians. They found "statistically significant improvement in patient perception and ratings of physician empathy."[5] In a 2011 study of patients with diabetes, researchers found that patients who had rated their doctors highly on empathy scores were most likely to have good control of both hemoglobin A1c and LDL cholesterol.[6]

Further, a 2012 study of baby boomers (those born between 1945 and 1960) presents an interesting finding from this increasingly large segment of the patient population. Of the 400 people surveyed, 86% said their patient experience would be better if the doctors talked to them about changing their behavior rather than immediately prescribing a drug.[7]

More recommendations gleaned from various organizations and studies can be found in the chart of Patient Satisfaction Tips on p. 75.

Other industries have seen a direct correlation between revenue and positive customer experience. Forrester Research estimates that above-average customer satisfaction scores can save health insurance plans significant revenue.[8] The same metrics are becoming more important to the bottom line of individual medical practices as well and will become more so as the government puts its trust in patient satisfaction scores as a reliable indicator of quality care.

In some respects, the future is already here. The era of the empowered consumer, where online interactivity has allowed them to take greater control over their lives, is an excellent example of this phenomenon.

A recent survey of 6,000 adults found that patient satisfaction is more important than price, especially in healthcare. In a report released in July 2012, PwC Health Research Institute compared consumer attitudes in banking, hospitality, airline and retail industries to their experiences and opinions in healthcare.[9]

PwC found consumers have similar expectations of healthcare as compared to other industries: convenience and speed.

But the differences are more telling. The survey showed that price is not a top inducement for choosing a healthcare provider. Only 8% of respondents ranked price as the primary driver of their decision, compared to 69% for leisure airline travel, 55% for retail, and even 50% for selecting a health insurer.

Instead, 42% of consumers surveyed ranked *personal experience* as the primary criteria in choosing a healthcare provider. Overall, the study found that 72% of consumers ranked the reputation of the healthcare provider and personal experience as the top drivers for choosing a provider.[9] Other important findings include:

- **Attitude of the health team matters.** PwC found that, when compared to banking and hospitality industries, staff attitude was twice as important in healthcare provider decisions.
- **Apologies are viewed positively.** Healthcare consumers said they would be willing to go back to a provider who apologizes.
- **"Ideal" experiences drive change.** More than one-third of consumers said they would change providers or insurance plans if the providers offered an "ideal experience," defined in the study as non-clinical aspects of care, such as "convenience, amenities, and customer service."[9]

Stephen Schimpff, MD, an internist, professor of medicine and public policy, former CEO of the University of Maryland Medical Center, and author of *The Future of Medicine—Megatrends in Healthcare* and *The Future of Health Care Delivery*, writes[10]:

"Consumerism is becoming—finally—more and more of a driver of change. Patients are coming to want and *expect* to be treated like a valued customer. Like the movie where he shouted "I can't take it anymore," now "the patient is no longer willing to be patient anymore." What do the patients want? They want service, good service. They increasingly understand that quality and safety are not ideal so they are looking for and expecting high levels of quality & safety. Perhaps the most important one of all is respect, respect for their person, confidentially, and the quality of their care. But also patients want convenience & responsiveness. They don't want to have to travel long distances, wait long times in the "waiting room," nor be put on indefinite telephone hold. They want interaction by email and other electronic methods. And finally, patients increasingly expect to have a closing the information gap—they expect the playing field between patient and doctor to be much more level in the future."

Vivian Lee, MD, MBA, the CEO of the University of Utah Health Care, the nation's first health center to publish its own patient satisfaction surveys online, writes that patient satisfaction should not be considered in isolation but in the "context of other important metrics of delivery-system performance, such as measures of access, quality, and costs of care." This transparency, she concludes, "has the power to change the culture of health care."[11]

TAKING CHARGE OF YOUR ONLINE PRESENCE

Given the importance of your online presence, it helps to know where you stand. Google yourself. You may find mixed results, some positive and some negative reviews. Most likely, the results of your Google search will be inconclusive. Most of the rating sites will contain basic data, such as where you went to medical school, years in practice, and the names of hospitals where you work. On some of the sites, that is all the information you will find. There may be a couple of reviews from patients, but many sites, will have no reviews at all.

If Google searches uncover so little information, why waste your time?

1. Establish a positive presence. Research data show that consumer use of the Internet to find and comment on their experiences with healthcare is growing. If you do not have many ratings now, consider yourself lucky that you're able to get in on the ground floor in establishing a positive online presence and cultivating positive reviews from your patients. Even your current patients may be watching!

Next year or the year after, when potential patients do a search and find several physicians' profiles that meet their criteria for specialty or geography, you don't want yours to be the profile with no information about your practice. A straightforward and positive online presence could boost your business now and in the future.

2. Correct errors and out-of-date information. Review sites pre-populate their listings with data that are readily available, such as your practice name and address. However, the information they have is not always correct. Maybe one physician left the practice and joined another. Maybe your office has moved. Sometimes the information is just completely wrong and there's no explanation.

The best way to combat incorrect information is to "claim" your business listing. Most rating sites allow physicians to manage their basic data. Once you are verified as the legitimate owner of the business, you will have complete control over the information the site shows about you and your practice. Do not neglect this step, as incorrect information can lead potential patients to the wrong address or directly to a competing practice. If you have moved to a new practice but the group you were previously with still exists, potential patients who call your old phone number will probably be offered an appointment with a doctor in that group. Most rating sites allow physicians to manage their basic data.

3. Read the reviews. Knowledge is power. No one wants their weaknesses broadcast to the whole world. Understandably, many healthcare professionals are nervous about the transparency brought about by social media, especially the trend toward online reviewing by patients. However, feedback can be healthy, allowing you to discover ways to improve patients' experiences with all aspects of your practice. Read the reviews and take them to heart.

4. Claim your identity. One fact of life in our increasingly small and interactive world is that there are no names that are truly unique to one person. No matter how unusual you think your name is, chances are there is at least one other person somewhere in the world with the same name and with an Internet presence who is *also* a healthcare professional!

Internist Vineet Arora, MD, associate program director of the University of Chicago's internal medicine residency program, tells what happened the first time she Googled herself.[12]

"My online reputation was not something I had ever thought of until I had a bad one. When someone would Google my name, he or she would find the top hits referred to my exact namesake, Vineet Arora, an ophthalmologist in Ontario, Canada. This would not be so terrible, except that most of the links were accompanied by a headline like "Ophthalmologist accused of blinding patients."

Needless to say, that really concerned me.

Would people think I was that guy? My name and even professional identity was associated with this other person. What's worse is that my own faculty profile at the University of Chicago was not coming up high in the search. So at that moment, I decided to generate my own online content.

The first thing I did was set up a LinkedIn account as a landing page for myself that included a list of my positions. I will confess that I was afraid of being too "out there" at first, so I kept my LinkedIn page pretty barebones.

I link all my social media accounts to my LinkedIn page. I also created a Google profile and a very cool page on About.me to aggregate Web content related to my work.

Controlling my online reputation allows me to control what people say about me, too. For example, when I give talks, I simply send my Google profile bio, as opposed to having someone reinvent the wheel from my CV.

I share my story with trainees so that they not only become familiar with their online reputation, but also take control of it. Even if they are not ready to dive fully into social media, setting up a LinkedIn page is an easy first step to building an online reputation.

Because I see patients only when they are hospitalized in an urban academic center that cares for an underserved, diverse population, my patients don't likely know who I am until they meet me. But these days, the minute you hear about someone you don't know, what do you do? You Google them. So I would not be surprised if that is what some of my patients do, and certainly more will do so in the future.

In this day and age, because your online reputation is often your first impression, it better be a good one."

FEAR NOT ONLINE RATINGS

Often, the topic of online ratings causes a sense of anxiety among physicians, as most have not been trained to deal with being reviewed online.

Many physicians say their greatest fear is Googling their name and seeing a negative review from one of these sites. What if, when you Google yourself, you were to find comments like these, taken from real reviews at a physician rating site:

"Going to this dermatologist was a waste of time and money."

"What a mistake. This man has the bedside manner of someone from the Amazon."

These comments were taken from real reviews at a physician rating site. It's obviously not how you want patients to find you on the Web.

Despite the damage bad reviews can do to your online reputation, there is tremendous value in social media, and the time it takes to develop a strong online reputation is time well-spent. If you want to determine the impact of social media on your practice, simply ask new patients how they found you. A growing percentage of are there because of information they found about you online.

Also, consider this: patients who've explored your practice online may also be more comfortable with you, because they may feel as though they already know you. They may be more willing to share their concerns because they've read an article or an interview about you. In addition, because they have made a conscious decision to come to you (perhaps even selected you from among several choices), they may be more receptive to your instructions. Not only might this enhanced comfort level make the relationship between you and your patient stronger, it could minimize the chance that the patient will go elsewhere after the initial visit.

MONITOR—YES. RESPOND? MAYBE, MAYBE NOT

Once you have an online presence, maintain your online reputation by monitoring online reviews as they appear. This should be an important part of your practice management agenda.

Set up a Google alert for your practice so that any time a review is posted, you should get a notice about it. When you set up the alert, be sure to include providers' names as well as the name of the practice so you are alerted whenever a review is posted about not only the practice, but also about individual providers.

Monitoring your profiles for reviews is always a good idea; responding to the reviews is another matter altogether. Medical professionals have different standards than other types of businesses that are reviewed online and some rules for reputation management don't apply to you!

For example, Yelp encourages businesses to "create a Yelp deal" by offering discounts to customers who find businesses on their site. They also advise business owners to message customers and join the conversation. None of these techniques is appropriate for the medical practice.

However, physicians have several options for responding to patient reviews that are consistent with professional standards.

How to respond to negative reviews

The good news is that studies have shown that most reviews of physicians are positive, but a negative review is inevitable. Online reputation companies often try to bury bad reviews by creating more positive information to improve the search rankings of a business. Some of their strategies include publishing numerous press releases with positive news about the business or individual, and creating multiple websites about various products and services of a business as a way to divert attention away from the negative reviews, and give it more positive visibility in search results. Most medical practices do not lend themselves to these types of solutions.

Doctors actually have numerous options for responding to patient reviews. Eric Goldman, professor of law at Santa Clara University School of Law has written extensively on legal issues relating to online rating sites and offers these suggestions[13]:

- **Respond generally.** Because most negative reviews relate to non-clinical aspects of the practice such as parking, wait times, out-of-date magazines or staff attitude, doctors can respond to those issues directly within the review site without violating privacy laws. Explain these aspects of your practice without confirming or denying that the reviewer was your patient. Explain how you run your practice in general terms, but refrain from publicly talking about the specifics of any one patient's experience.

- **Address individuals offline.** Responding to negative reviews that criticize bedside manner or question medical judgment should *never* be done in a public forum. Some sites, like Yelp, allow providers to privately respond to patient reviews. You may take the opportunity to do so. But it's better to take this conversation offline. An invitation to call the office to further discuss the concern is appropriate.

- **Ask for permission to reply.** Finally, you can ask patients for their permission to publicly reply to their reviews, or post an apology. Once you have their written consent, a public response or apology can show others in the forum that you are listening to patients and taking steps to address their concerns. This may turn the negative situation into a more constructive experience.[14]

Posting responses is reactive and shouldn't be your only strategy for combating negative reviews. Those reviews will live a long time online, and could become fodder for malpractice attorneys or could impact your ability to sell your practice.

Instead, be proactive. Consider the patient's experience and make sure the customer service aspects of your practice meet acceptable standards as part of the new definition of professionalism in medicine. Once you excel in service, encourage more patients to review you online. In the end, any negative reviews will appear to be outliers.

At the end of the day, a negative review is inevitable. Here's something else to think about: Many people believe that, if you have a number of ratings, and only one or two are negative, the ratings overall may be perceived as more credible than if they were uniformly glowing reviews![14]

Lawsuits are not the answer

Most rating sites listed in this book have procedures to remove negative reviews if they are found to be fraudulent or otherwise violate a site's Terms of Service. But the burden of proof rests largely with the doctor. Fighting a negative review can take months of gathering information and negotiating with the ratings site before any action is taken. Unless they find a specific policy violation or fraud, they are unlikely to remove a negative review because doing so would infringe on a patient's right to free speech.

Some healthcare providers have gone to court over negative ratings that they believe are unfair. This practice is generally not recommended because a lawsuit is not likely to produce a successful outcome. In addition, it is extremely time-consuming and expensive.

As an alternative, doctors and medical facilities have started suing patients to have negative reviews removed—and some have done so successfully. These doctors often have legal teams and the necessary funding to support their fight, so the threat of a suit can be enough to compel the patient to remove a negative review.[15]

You must establish that untrue statements were made as fact and that those statements hurt your reputation. Reviews are usually opinions, making defamation suits hard to win. You must establish that untrue statements were made as fact and that those statements hurt your reputation. What's worse, the case could create a media firestorm in your community or on a regional or national level, depending on the circumstances of the case. An attempt to censor or remove information online may backfire and instead of being deleted, the information may be shared across the Internet in a very short time. This was the case when Barbra Streisand filed a lawsuit over the online posting of an aerial photo of her house—leading the phenomenon to be known as the Streisand Effect—an attempt to censor or remove information online backfires and the opposite actually occurs. Instead of being deleted, the situation gets widespread publicity and is often shared across the Internet in a very short timeframe.

Regardless what kind of merit you think a case might have, doctors who sue patients for online ratings are going to lose in the more influential court of public opinion. Better that doctors take some slanderous lumps online and instead encourage more of their patients to rate them. The ensuing positive ratings will drown out any vitriol, making them outliers.

However, resist the temptation to broadcast your positive reviews with abandon. HIPAA rules give patients complete control over how and where their protected health information is used and this law includes anything they write online about their healthcare experiences. In 2016, a physical therapy practice was fined by a California health agency for posting patient testimonials on its website without the express permission of the patients! If you would like to quote from any reviews you find online, you must get permission first.[16]

ECONOMICS OF GOOD REVIEWS

Research from Harvard suggests there is a real bottom-line benefit to cultivating positive online reviews. The study showed that where Yelp reviews were prevalent in a local market, chain restaurant business declined as consumers gained confidence about the quality of smaller, local restaurants.[17] This has implications for independent practices in that it may mean that there is an opportunity for small practices to compete against urgent care clinics, hospitals, and other large entities by using an effective online review strategy. It's a simple and cost-effective way to reach and recruit new patients. The same survey also found that a one-star rating increase could be directly tied to up to a 9% increase in revenue for a small business—another finding that may have implications for healthcare providers.

The other economic benefit of positive online reviews is that it helps the practice maintain overall high ranking in online search results. When reviews are combined with a strong social media presence, good search engine optimization, and an effective website, your practice can quickly rise to the top of the leading search engines like Google, driving traffic back to your website and more patients to your practice.[18]

The study by Software Advice show that a significant percentage of patients are willing to overlook important factors, such as cost inconvenience, in favor of positive online reviews. Their survey shows that 48% of patients are willing to go out of network for a doctor who has positive reviews and researchers predict that this percentage will grow.[3]

CORRELATION WITH CLINICAL OUTCOMES

Many physicians wonder how ratings are tied to quality, or even if they can be. After all, there is great variability in the number of reviews and, in fact, in the number of patients or procedures performed among doctors. Add to that the subjective nature of the review process and the different metrics across review sites and the picture gets even cloudier.

Evidence in the medical literature indicates there are positive correlations between patient satisfaction ratings and clinical outcomes.

A 2004 study by researchers at Press Ganey looked at inpatient ratings for patients hospitalized for five common conditions: heart attack, heart failure, stroke, pneumonia, and childbirth. Although patients with different conditions expressed different levels of satisfaction and had different care needs, this study found that patients who believed that their values and preferences were respected and that they had good emotional support from healthcare professionals had better outcomes. The researchers concluded that "good communication between patients and care providers drives positive patient experiences and compliance, which led to positive outcomes."[18]

A 2010 study examined the relationship between patient satisfaction and adherence to practice guidelines and outcomes for acute myocardial infarction. Researchers used clinical data on 6,467 patients treated at 25 U.S. hospitals, and cardiac patient satisfaction surveys from 3,562 patients treated at the same hospitals during the same time period. Higher patient satisfaction scores were associated with lower inpatient mortality, even after controlling for a hospital's overall guideline adherence score.[19]

Another study in 2007 looked at the relationship between patient perceptions of hospital practices and infection rates in 87 Pennsylvania hospitals. The authors found that facilities with higher patient satisfaction scores on cleanliness, blood-draw skills, and nurse responsiveness tended to also have lower rates of infection and infection mortality.[20]

However, not all published studies reach positive conclusions about patient ratings as they relate to clinical outcomes. A study from the *Archives of Internal Medicine* gives credence to some physicians' concerns that obtaining good ratings means giving in to patients' demands. According to the study, compared to the least-satisfied patients, those who were most satisfied with their healthcare were on more prescription medications, made more doctor's office visits, and were more likely to have had one or more hospital stays, despite the fact they were in better overall physical and mental health. Also, despite the greater attention and all those prescription drugs they got, the highly satisfied were more likely to die in the few years after taking the survey than were those who pronounced themselves least satisfied with their physicians' medical care.[21]

The authors of one study attempt to explain some of the differences in study findings pertaining to outcomes. Manary and colleagues reported in the *New England Journal of Medicine* that studies have shown that patient-experience measures are not positively correlated with an increase in services ordered. In fact, they lead to decreased use of resources while at the same time greater patient satisfaction.[22]

The authors further maintain that some studies with negative associations between patient satisfaction measures and outcomes only looked at communication between the patient and his/her physician. Limiting patient-experience measurement to a single dimension may exclude the interactions that most strongly affect experiences and outcomes.

Overall, they conclude that despite methodological issues, patient-experience surveys are good indicators of healthcare quality, and that the focus should be on how to improve patient experiences found to be associated with both satisfaction and outcomes.[22]

Beyond the impact of online reviews on patient outcomes is the broader issue of the effect social media can have on patients' health. Mediabistro found that 40% of consumers say that information found via social media affects the way they deal with their health.[23] They also found a big generational difference: 18- to 24-year-olds are more than twice as likely than 45- to 54-year-olds to use social media for health-related discussions.

Furthermore, a study by Search Engine Watch showed that consumers in the 18–24 age group said they would trust information shared by others on their social media networks.[23] But we all know that not all information found there is reliable or accurate! Thus, it's up to healthcare professionals to create and link to educational content that can be used and shared by patients for the betterment of their health.

As the famous line from *Field of Dreams* advises, if you build it they will come. Studies have shown that consumers want and respect the opinions of physicians.

Overall, sharing health-related information, whether it is with other consumers or one's doctor, is improving the way people feel about transparency and authenticity, which could lead to more productive discussions regarding a patient's health. In fact, one study showed that 60% of doctors believe that the transparency of social media is improving the quality of care provided to patients.[23] All healthcare professionals should ensure that they are part of these conversations.

Patient Satisfaction Tips

1. Understand your patients' preferences. Do they want phone calls, e-mails, or texts for appointment reminders? Adjust your communications practices accordingly.
2. Focus solutions on transparency, knowledge, and convenience. Consider offering mobile check-in, digital appointment reminders, medical reminders, price comparison tools, and free Wi-Fi.
3. Take advantage of multiple access points to educate and engage consumers. Provide in-person customer support for those who prefer it and virtual support for people who prefer that approach.
4. Train staff to welcome each patient with a smile, declutter the front desk, refrain from having food and beverages in sight, keep personal conversations quiet and to a minimum, and dress appropriately for the office.
5. Grant employees authority to change the customer experience. Train all staff on how to talk to patients, review staff performance, and share stories to improve the patient experience.
6. Don't keep patients waiting more than 15 minutes. If you are running behind schedule, consider sending patients a text message to alert them.
7. Talk to patients about behavioral changes they can make to improve their health.
8. Be proactive—go beyond the transaction. Train staff to acknowledge difficult situations and apologize.
9. Give patients a printed summary of their visit, including diagnosis and action plans.
10. Communication is key—make eye contact, involve patients in discussions of treatment options, and express complex information in layman's terms.
11. Keep the office environment attractive—have current and diverse magazines, clean furniture, healthy plants, straightened pictures and posters, music or TV that is not too loud, and clean restrooms.
12. Seek customer feedback.

Source: Pho K, Gay S. Patient Satisfaction Tips. *Establishing, Managing, and Protecting Your Online Reputation: A Social Media Guide for Physicians and Medical Practices.* 2013, Greenbranch Publishing

REFERENCES

1. PwC Health Research Institute. Scoring healthcare. New York: PriceWaterhouseCoopers U.S., 2013. https://www.beckershospitalreview.com/quality/study-healthcare-reviews-ratings-increasingly-impact-hospitals-bottom-lines.html.

2. King R.H., Stanley, J. and Baum, N. Hard internet truths: 34,748 online reviews reveal what patients really want from doctors. *J Med Pract Manage.* 2016; 1(5):309-12.

3. Loria, G. How patients use online reviews. Software Advice. 2018. https://www.softwareadvice.com/resources/how-patients-use-online-reviews/ Accessed August 2, 2018.

4. Anderson R., Barbara A., and Feldman S. What patients want: A content analysis of key qualities that influence patient satisfaction. *J Med Pract Manage. 2007; 22:255-61.*

5. Reiss H. Teaching empathy can improve patient satisfaction. *Vital Signs.* Massachusetts Medical Society. October 2012; http://www.massmed.org/News-and-Publications/Vital-Signs/Back-Issues/Teaching-Empathy-Can-Improve-Patient-Satisfaction/#.W2M6jdhKi_o. Accessed August 2, 2018.

6. Hojat M., Louis D.Z., Markham F.W., et al. Physicians' empathy and clinical outcomes for diabetic patients. *Acad Med. 2011; 86:359-64.*

7. Catalyst Healthcare Research. *Innovative ways to improve the patient experience.* Nashville: Catalyst Healthcare Research, 2012.

8. Forrester Research. *The business impact of customer experience,* 2012. Cambridge, MA: Forrester, 2012.

9. PwC Health Research Institute. Customer experience in healthcare: The moment of truth. New York: PriceWaterhouseCoopers U.S., July 2012.

10. Schimpff S. Disruptive changes are coming to the delivery system. *KevinMD Blog.* April 2, 2012; www.kevinmd.com/blog/2012/04/disruptive-coming-delivery-system.html. Accessed August 2, 2018.

11. Lee V. Transparency and trust—online patient reviews of physicians. *N Engl J Med.* 2017; 376:197-99.

12. Aurora V. from *Establishing, Managing, and Protecting Your Online Reputation.* Phoenix, MD: Greenbranch Publishing, 2013, pp. 30-32.

13. Goldman E. Doctors' online reputation management and patient reviews. *Technology & Marketing Law Blog.* May 21, 2012. http://blog.ericgoldman.org/archives/2012/05/doctors_online.htm. Accessed August 2, 2018.

14. Segal J. Managing your online reputation. *J Med Pract Manage.* 2012; 27(6): 341-43.

15. Scotti A. Some doctors are suing patients for posting negative reviews about their care online. *NY Daily News,* July 18, 2018. http://www.nydailynews.com/news/national/ny-news-doctors-suing-patients-online-reviews-20180718-story.html. Accessed August 2, 2018.

16. Minc A. How doctors can respond to negative online reviews—without breaking the law or calling further attention to criticisms. Minclaw Blog. January 5, 2018. https://www.minclaw.com/how-doctors-can-respond-to-negative-online-reviews/. Accessed August 2, 2018.

17. Luca M. Reviews, reputation, and revenue: the case of Yelp.com. Cambridge, MA: Harvard Business School, 2011. https://www.hbs.edu/faculty/Publication%20Files/12-016_a7e4a5a2-03f9-490d-b093-8f951238dba2.pdf Accessed August 2, 2018.

18. Gesell S.B., and Wolosin, R.J. Inpatients' ratings of care in 5 common clinical conditions. *Qual Manag Health Care.* 2004; 13:222-27.

19. Glickman S.W., Boulding W., Manary M., et al. Patient satisfaction and its relationship with clinical quality and inpatient mortality in acute myocardial infarction. *Circ Cardiovasc Qual Outcomes.* 2010; 3:188-95.

20. Trucano M., Kaldenberg D. The relationship between patient perceptions of hospital practices and facility infection rates: evidence from Pennsylvania hospitals. *Patient Safety & Quality Healthcare,* 2007.

21. Fenton J.J., Jerant A.F., Bertakis K.D., and Franks P. The cost of satisfaction: a national study of patient satisfaction, health care utilization, expenditures, and mortality. *Archives of Internal Medicine.* 2012;172(5):405-11.

22. Manary M.P., Boulding W., Staelin R., and Clickman S. The patient experience and health outcomes. *N Engl J Med.* 2013; 368:201-03.

23. Honigman B. 24 Outstanding statistics & figures on how social media has impacted the healthcare industry. Referral MD. 2013. https://getreferralmd.com/2013/09/healthcare-social-media-statistics/. Accessed August 2, 2018.

Template Gallery

Appendix 1

BUSINESS ASSOCIATE AGREEMENT

This Business Associate Agreement (this "Agreement") is entered into this _____ day of _____ 20___, by and between (PROVIDER NAME) (Covered Entity") and (COMPANY NAME) ("Business Associate").

RECITALS

A. Covered Entity is a Covered Entity under the Health Insurance Portability and Accountability Act ("HIPAA") and Health Information Technology for Economic and Clinical Health Act ("HITECH") and as such must comply with the Administrative Simplification Provisions of HIPAA, including the Privacy Standards (as defined in Article 1 of this Agreement), as of the dates indicated in instructions from the relevant federal agencies.

B. Covered Entity is interested in Business Associate furnishing (DESCRIBE SERVICES TO BE PROVIDED) to Covered Entity and Business Associate has the expertise necessary to provide such services.

C. In order for Business Associate to furnish services to Covered Entity in accordance with this Business Associate Agreement, Covered Entity intends to disclose certain Protected Health Information (hereinafter "PHI") (as defined in Article 1 of this Agreement) of Covered Entity patients to Business Associate and expects Business Associate to use the PHI to perform its obligations under the Agreement.

D. Business Associate is a "Business Associate" within the meaning of the Privacy Standards and federal law.

E. Covered Entity will not transfer PHI to a Business Associate or permit the Business Associate to receive PHI on behalf of Covered Entity without satisfactory assurances from the Business Associate that it will appropriately safeguard the information.

F. Business Associate desires to provide the satisfactory assurances required by the Privacy Standards and further define the Parties' rights and responsibilities for the exchange of PHI.

NOW, THEREFORE, the Parties, in consideration of the mutual agreements herein contained and for other good and valuable consideration, the receipt and adequacy of which are hereby acknowledged, do hereby agree as follows:

ARTICLE 1: DEFINITIONS

1.1   **Definitions.** For the purposes of this Agreement, the following defined terms shall have the following definitions.

    a. **"Designated Record Set"** shall mean a group of records maintained by or for Covered Entity that is (i) the medical records and billing records about individuals maintained by or for Covered Entity, and (ii) used, in whole or in part, by or for Covered Entity to make decisions about individuals. For the purposes of this paragraph, the term "Record" means any items, collection, or grouping of information that includes PHI and is maintained, collected, used, or disseminated by or for Covered Entity.

    b. **"HHS"** shall mean the United States Department of Health and Human Services.

    c. **"Individually Identifiable Health Information"** shall mean information that is a subset of health information, including demographic information collected from an individual, as defined in 45 C.F.R. § 164.501 of the Privacy Standards.

    d. **"Privacy Standards"** shall mean the Standards for Privacy of Individually Identifiable Health Information found at 45 C.F.R. §§ 160 and 164.

    e. **"Protected Health Information"** shall mean, certain Individually Identifiable Health Information, as defined in 45 C.F.R. § 164.501 of the Privacy Standards.

    f. **"Secretary"** shall mean the Secretary of HHS.

ARTICLE 2: PERMITTED USES AND DISCLOSURES
BY BUSINESS ASSOCIATE

2.1   **Purpose.** Business Associate's role is to provide **(DESCRIPTION OF SERVICES/ DUTIES)** to the Covered Entity.

2.2   **Disclosure of PHI.**

    a. Business Associate may only use or disclose PHI in the course and scope of its actions on behalf of Covered Entity.

    b. Business Associate may use or disclose PHI as required by law.

    c. Business Associate agrees to make use and disclosures and request for PHI consistent with covered entities minimum necessary policies and procedures.

    d. Business Associate may not use or disclose PHI in a manner that would violate sub part E of 45CFR Part 164 if done by Covered Entity.

    e. Business Associate may use protected PHI for proper management and administration of Business Associate to carry out legal responsibilities of the Business Associate, provided the disclosures are required by law, or Business Associate 1) obtains reasonable assurance from person to whom the information is disclosed that the information will remain confidential and be used or further disclosed only as required by law or for purposes for which it was disclosed to the person, 2) the person notifies Business Associate of any instances of which it is aware in which the confidentiality of the information has been breached, and 3) PHI remains within the jurisdiction of HHS at all times.

    f. Business Associate may provide data aggregation services related to health care operations of the Covered Entity.

ARTICLE 3: DUTIES OF BUSINESS ASSOCIATE

3.1   **Disclosures.** Business Associate shall not disclose PHI other than as permitted or required by this Agreement or as required by law.

3.2   **Safeguards.** Business Associate shall use appropriate safeguards, comply with subpart C of CFR Part 164 with respect to electronic PHI, to prevent use or disclosure of PHI other than as provided for by this Agreement.

3.3   **Reporting of Unauthorized Disclosure or Use.** Business Associate shall report to Covered Entity any use or disclosure of PHI not provided for by this Agreement of which it becomes aware including breaches of unsecured PHI as required by 45 CFR 164.410. Further, Business Associate shall report any security incident of which it becomes aware that involves Covered Entity's PHI to Covered Entity. All reporting required under this provision (3.3), shall be made by Business Associate within ten (10) business days of first awareness of the issue. Any use of disclosure of PHI not provided for by this Agreement shall be reported pursuant to 6.3 below **and** by telephone to (TELEPHONE NUMBER) or email to (EMAIL ADDRESS).

3.4   **Subcontractors.** Business Associate in accordance with 45 CFR 164.502(e) I (ii) and 164.380(b)(ii) ensure that any subcontractors that create, receive, maintain, or transmit PHI on behalf of the Business Associate agree to the same restrictions, conditions, and requirements that apply to the Business Associate under this Agreement and under federal law.   Further, subcontractors must keep all PHI within the jurisdiction of HHS.

3.5   **Designated Records Set.** Business Associate shall make available PHI and a Designated Record Set to the Covered Entity as is necessary to satisfy Covered Entity's obligations under 45 CFR 164.524.

3.6   **Amendments to PHI.** Business Associate shall make any amendment(s) to PHI in a designated record set as directed or agreed to by the Covered Entity pursuant to 45 CFR 164.526, or take other measures as are necessary to satisfy Covered Entity's obligations under 45 CFR 164.526.

3.7   **Accounting of Disclosures.** Business Associate shall maintain and make available information required to provide an accounting of disclosures to the Covered Entity as is necessary to satisfy the Covered Entity's obligation under 45 CFR 164.528.

3.8   **Performance of Covered Entities Obligation.** In the event Business Associate is to carry out one or more of Covered Entity's obligations under Subpart E of 45 CFR 164, Business Associate shall comply with the requirements of Subpart E that comply to the Covered Entity in the performance of such obligation(s).

3.9   **Documentation Availability.** Business Associate shall make its internal practices, policies, books, security risk analysis reports, breach log and records (whether they be in electronic, magnetic, or on paper) available to the Secretary and to Covered Entity for purposes of determining compliance with the HIPAA rules.

3.10 **Employees of Business Associate.** Business Associate shall make reasonable efforts to ensure that its employees have not been convicted of any felony or been dishonorably discharge from military service. Further, Business Associate agrees that Covered Entity may immediately terminate all contractual relationships, including by not limited to, this Agreement if Business Associate employs, or utilizes any convicted felon in furtherance of this Agreement.

3.11 **Agents of Business Associate.** Business Associate may not, without prior written consent of Covered Entity, outsource, subcontract, refer or otherwise transfer PHI of Covered Entity to any third party.

3.12 **Audit.** Covered Entity may, upon reasonable notice to Business Entity, audit and/or review physically or remotely, Business Entity's information technology systems and facilities. Any costs associated with an audit shall be the sole responsibility of Covered Entity.

3.13 Business Associate may not, without prior written consent of Covered Entity, post or submit information or questions to any electronic form (list serves, discussion boards, etc.) that in any way reference Covered Entity or Covered Entity's PHI.

3.14 Business Associate may not, without prior written consent of Covered Entity (or as required by law) make any reference to Covered Entity or Covered Entity's PHI on any website or social media site.

ARTICLE 4: TERM AND TERMINATION

4.1 **Basic Term.** The Term of this Agreement shall be effective as of the above stated date, and shall terminate when all of the Protected Health Information provided by Covered Entity to Business Associate, or created or received by Business Associate on behalf of Covered Entity, is destroyed or returned to Covered Entity, or, if it is infeasible to return or destroy Protected Health Information, protections are extended to such information, in accordance with the termination provisions of this Section.

4.2 **Termination for Material Breach.** A material breach of this Agreement which is not addressed within thirty (30) days of written notice by the Covered Entity is grounds for termination by the Business Associate. Covered Entity may elect to terminate this Agreement immediately upon written notice to Business Associate where Business Associate commits a material breach.

ARTICLE 5: INDEMNIFICATION

5.1 Business Associate hereby saves and holds Covered Entity harmless of and from, and indemnifies and agrees to defend it against any and all losses, liability, damages and expenses (including, without limitation, reasonable attorney's fees and expenses) which Covered Entity may incur or be compelled to pay, or for which Covered Entity may become liable or compelled to pay in any action, claim, or proceeding against Covered Entity, its officers, directors, employees, agents, or servants, for or by reason of any acts, whether of omission or commission, that may be committed or suffered by Covered Entity or any of its officers, directors, employees, agents, or servants in connection with Business Associate's performance of its obligations under this Agreement and/or the Privacy Standards.

5.2 This Section shall survive termination of this Agreement.

ARTICLE 6: GENERAL PROVISIONS

6.1 The Parties expressly acknowledge that it is, and shall continue to be, their intent to fully comply with all relevant federal, state, and local laws, rules, and regulations.

6.2 This Agreement shall be governed in all respects, whether as to validity, construction, capacity, performance or otherwise, by the laws of the State of **(WHERE PRACTICE IS)**, notwithstanding any conflict of interest rules that might otherwise apply.

6.3 All notices or communications required or permitted pursuant to the terms of this Agreement shall be in writing and will be delivered in person or by means of certified or registered mail, postage paid, return receipt requested, to such Party at its address as set forth below, or such other person or address as such Party may specify by similar notice to the other Party hereto, or by telephone facsimile with a hard copy sent by mail with delivery on the next business day. All such notices will be deemed given upon delivery or delivered by hand, on the third business day after deposit with the U.S. Postal Service, and on the first business day after sending if by facsimile.

As to Covered Entity:

> COMPANY NAME & ADDRESS)
> (Telephone)
> Attn: **(Office Manager/Privacy Officer)**

As to Business Associate:

> (COMPANY NAME & ADDRESS)
> (Telephone)
> Attn: (NAME)

6.4 This Agreement, including any exhibits attached hereto, constitutes the entire Agreement among the Parties hereto with respect to their respective obligations for compliance with the HIPAA Privacy Standards and supersedes any and all prior agreements or statements among the Parties hereto, both oral and written, concerning the subject matter hereof. This Agreement may supplement any other agreements between the Parties. This Agreement may not be amended, modified or terminated except by a writing signed by both Parties.

6.5 If any provision of this Agreement shall be held invalid or unenforceable, such invalidity or unenforceability shall attach only to such provision and shall not in any way affect or render invalid or unenforceable any other provision of this Agreement.

6.6 The waiver by either Party of a breach or violation of any provision of this Agreement shall not operate as, or be construed to be, a waiver of any subsequent breach of the same or other provisions of this Agreement.

6.7 This Agreement may be executed in any number of counterparts, all of which together shall constitute one and the same instrument.

6.8 This Agreement shall be binding upon and inure to the benefit of the Parties hereto and their respective successors and assigns. Neither Party shall assign or delegate its rights, duties, or obligations under this Agreement, without the prior written consent of the other Party.

6.9 In the performance of the duties and obligations of the Parties pursuant to this Agreement, each of the Parties shall at all times be acting and performing as an independent contractor, and nothing in this Agreement shall be construed or deemed to create a relationship of employer and employee, or partner, or joint venture, or principal and agent between the Parties.

6.10 A reference in this Agreement to a section in the Privacy Standards means the section as in effect or as amended.

6.11 The Parties agree to take such action as is necessary to amend this Agreement from time to time as is necessary for the Parties to comply with the requirements of the Privacy Standards.

6.12 Individually executing this Agreement on behalf of a Party, acknowledge and represent that the individual has the legal authority to contractually bind the Party he or she is signing on behalf of.

IN WITNESS WHEREOF, the Parties hereto have affixed their hands and seals on the day and date first above written.

_____ **. by**   _____ **(Business Associate) by**
(Name and Title)   (Name and Title)

Appendix 2

POP UP-NOTICE ON WEBSITE PRIOR TO A PATIENT COMMUNICATING WITH YOUR OFFICE

To Our Patients:

By choosing to use email to communicate with us, you understand and agree to the following: The use of email poses risks to the confidentiality of your health information. The Internet is an open network and provides no inherent protection for confidential information. You accept these risks and waive the requirements under the HITECH Act for us to communicate with you. Further, email sent to our office may not be routinely monitored. Please contact our practice by telephone (**TELEPHONE #**) or in person about critical or time-sensitive issues. In the event of a medical emergency, please contact 911.

Notice on bottom of emails:

Notice: This email and any files transmitted with it are confidential and covered by the Electronic Communications Privacy Act and are intended solely for the use of the individual or entity to whom they are addressed. Any protected health information (PHI) contained in the email is HIGHLY CONFIDENTIAL. It is to be used only to aid in providing specific healthcare services to this patient. Any other use is a violation of federal law (HIPAA) and will be reported as such. If you are not the intended recipient or the individual responsible for delivering the email to the intended recipient, please be advised that you have received this email in error and that any use, dissemination, forwarding, printing, or copying of this email is strictly prohibited. If you have received this email in error, please immediately notify the sender and delete it. Thank you.

Notice on bottom of faxes:

Notice: This facsimile and any files transmitted with it are confidential and covered by the Electronic Communications Privacy Act and are intended solely for the use of the individual or entity to whom they are addressed. Any protected health information (PHI) contained in this facsimile is HIGHLY CONFIDENTIAL. It is to be used only to aid in providing specific healthcare services to this patient. Any other use is a violation of federal law (HIPAA) and will be reported as such. If you are not the intended recipient or the individual responsible for delivering the facsimile to the intended recipient, please be advised that you have received this facsimile in error and that any use, dissemination, scanning, or copying of this facsimile is strictly prohibited. If you have received this facsimile in error, please immediately notify the sender and shred it. Thank you.

Appendix 3

TERMS OF USE FOR THIS WEBSITE

Effective: _____

Welcome

Welcome to **(PRACTICE NAME)**'s website. We are pleased you are here. Please review carefully our "Terms of Use for This Website." These terms apply throughout our entire website. Additional terms may apply via state and federal laws. We hope you find our website useful.

I.   Note the Practice of Medicine

No website can replace the physician/patient relationship. Our website is designed to provide information about our practice and to offer useful information about healthcare issues. This website ***does not***:

- Establish a care provider/patient relationship.
- Provide specific medical advice.
- Constitute the practice of medicine.
- Provide a substitute for medical care.

Users of this website should always seek the advice of a licensed physician or other qualified healthcare provider with any questions regarding personal health or medical conditions. If you believe you have a medical problem or condition, please seek medical attention from a qualified provider.

*** If you believe you are experiencing a medical emergency, call 911 immediately.

II.   No Endorsements

Links from this website to third-party websites do <u>not</u> imply this practice's endorsement of any other websites' product or service. Links from this website to third-party websites are provided for your convenience and are intended only to enable access to these third-party websites and for <u>no</u> other purpose. Please use your independent caution and judgment when accessing these third-party websites.

III.   Designed and Operated for Adult Users

This website is designed and operated for users 18 years old and older; it is not intended to be accessed by children. Those under the age of 18 should have a parent or guardian assist with use of this website.

By using this website, you agree that you will not:

- Disrupt, disable, "hack" or in any way interfere with the proper functioning of this website.
- Use this website in a way that violates any law, act, or treaty.
- Copy or "scrape" any content or images from this website without this practice's prior written approval.

IV.   Secured Use of this Website

If you access our Patient Portal or any other secured access area of this website, you are responsible for maintaining the confidentiality of your account and password. You also are responsible for all activities and actions that are transacted under your account or password.

V.   Copyright Notice

You may not copy, reproduce, republish, repurpose, post, "scrape," or use in any way the content or images contained in this website without this practice's prior written approval.

VI.   Digital Millenium Copyright Act

This practice complies with the provisions of the Digital Millenium Copyright Act. If you have a concern regarding the use of copyrighted material on this website, please contact us at: (EMAIL ADDRESS).

VII. Disclaimers

You understand and agree that this practice's website and any services, content, or information contained on or provided by this practice are provided on an "as-is" basis. This practice does not make any express or implied warranties. In addition, this practice does not guarantee that use of its website will be free from technological difficulties including, but not limited to, unavailability of information, downtime, service disruptions, and viruses or worms. You understand that you are responsible for implementing sufficient procedures and checkpoints to satisfy your particular requirements for accuracy of data input and output.

VIII. Limitations of Liability

You assume any and all risks when using this website. This practice shall not be liable for any direct, indirect, consequential, monetary, punitive, special, or exemplary damages, fines, fees, or penalties that are in any way related to the use of this website.

Your sole and exclusive remedy for any claim or alleged claim arising from the use of this website is to STOP USING THIS WEBSITE.

[Please note that some states do not allow the limitation or exclusion of damages and/or liability. This means the above limitation of liability may not apply to your use of this website.]

IX.   Indemnification

You agree that you will indemnify and hold harmless this practice from any damages, losses, liabilities, judgments, costs, and/or expenses (including reasonable attorney fees) that in any way relate to your use or misuse of this website. This shall include any third-party claims that may arise as a consequence of your use of this website.

X.   Changes to this "Terms of Use for This Website" Statement

This practice may alter, modify, revise, or amend any or all of this "Terms of Use for this Website" at any time. Such alterations, modifications, revisions, or amendments shall be effective immediately upon either posting it/them to this website or upon notifying you.

XI.   Jurisdiction

You agree and consent that any claim or dispute that in any way relates to your use of this website is subject to the exclusive jurisdiction of (INSERT YOUR STATE). This consent and agreement also applies to any person attempting to advance a claim on your behalf.

XII.   Contacting Us

If you or anyone on your behalf has a question or concern about the "Terms of Use for this Website," please contact us at (EMAIL ADDRESS). Thank you.

Appendix 4

(PRACTICE NAME) SECURITY POLICY

Effective Date:

Approved By: (Title/Name of Board)

Issued By: (NAME), Compliance Officer

I.   Introduction

(PRACTICE NAME) pursuant to the Health Insurance Portability and Accountability Act (HIPAA) law and regulations is required to take reasonable steps to ensure the privacy of your Electronic Protected Health Information (ePHI). Protected Health Information (PHI) is individually identifiable health information related to the past, present, or future physical or mental health or condition of an individual; provision of healthcare to an individual; or the past, present, or future payment for the provision of healthcare to an individual. ePHI is any PHI that is created, accessed, transmitted, or received electronically. The HIPAA Security Rule provides for administrative, technical, and physical safeguards to ensure the confidentiality, integrity, and availability of all ePHI data that a covered component creates, receives, maintains, or transmits, and that such data is protected from unauthorized access, or loss.

II.   Scope of Policy

This policy is specific to the HIPAA Security Rule and applies only to those HIPAA-covered components identified in the Privacy Policy. All employees, staff members, and independent contractors of (PRACTICE NAME) are expected to fully comply with this policy. Additionally, all employees, staff, and independent contractors are expected to adhere to state and federal laws and regulations and to the (PRACTICE NAME) policies and procedures. Any employee, staff member, or independent contractor who disregards these policies and procedures, and/or related state or federal laws and regulations *will be subject to disciplinary action up to and including termination.*

III.   Administrative Safeguards

A. Risk Analysis

A yearly risk analysis will be performed on all covered components to identify the potential risks and vulnerabilities of ePHI maintained or transmitted electronically. This will include documentation of all repositories (whether temporary or permanent) of ePHI as well as allowed users of each repository. The risk analysis is to be presented to the Compliance Officer who will identify remedial steps for identified risks. [HIPAA Section 164.308 (a)(1)]

B. Risk Management

All covered components will implement measures to reduce computer risks and vulnerabilities, including identifying and documenting potential risks and vulnerabilities that could impact systems managing ePHI; performing annual technical security assessments of systems managing ePHI in order to identify and remedy detected security vulnerabilities. [Addresses HIPAA Section 164.308(a)(1).]

C. Sanctions

Any employee or staff member who fails to comply with HIPAA laws and regulations, state or other federal privacy laws, or (PRACTICE NAME)'s Security Policy and procedures will be subject to disciplinary action and sanctions commensurate with the gravity of the violation. Such violations may include, but are not limited to, re-training, verbal and written warnings, temporary suspension without pay, or termination. The (PRACTICE NAME) will investigate any potential HIPAA security violation or incident in a timely manner. The (PRACTICE NAME) will not intimidate, threaten, coerce, discriminate against, or take any retaliation against any employee who reports a HIPAA security violation or incident. [See HIPAA Section 164.308(a)(1).]

D. Information System Activity Review

All covered components will periodically review information system activity records—including audit logs, access reports, and security incident tracking reports—to ensure that implemented security controls are effective and that ePHI has not been potentially compromised. [Addresses HIPAA Section 164.308(a)(1).] Measures should include:

1. Enabling logging on computer systems managing ePHI.
2. Developing a process for the review of exception reports and/or logs.
3. Developing and documenting procedures for the retention of monitoring data. Log information should be maintained for up to six years, either locally on the server or through the use of backup tapes.
4. Periodically reviewing compliance to the (PRACTICE NAME)'s Information Security Policy and its associated procedures.

E. Assigned Security Responsibility

(PRACTICE NAME) has appointed a Compliance Officer to ensure compliance with the HIPAA. The Compliance Officer is responsible for the development and implementation of policies, procedures, and training programs that will ensure compliance with the HIPAA Security Rule. The Compliance Officer may delegate some or all of the responsibilities in carrying out the requirements of this policy. [HIPAA Section 164.208 (a)(2)]

F. Workforce Security

All covered components will establish procedures that ensure only authorized personnel have access to systems that manage ePHI. [Addresses HIPAA Section 164.308(a)(3).] Measures that each covered component should address include:

1. Establishing a procedure that requires managerial approval before any person is granted access to systems managing ePHI.
2. Performing background checks, where appropriate, before any person is granted access to systems managing ePHI.
3. Limiting authorized persons' access to ePHI to the extent that access to this information achieves the requirements of the person's job responsibilities.
4. Implementing procedures for terminating access to ePHI when the employment of a person ends or the job responsibilities of the person no longer warrant access to ePHI.
5. Periodically reviewing the accounts on systems managing ePHI to ensure that only currently authorized persons have access to these systems.

G. Information Access Management

Each covered component will establish procedures to assign, implement, revoke, and modify access to ePHI. [HIPAA 164.308(a)(4)

H. Security Awareness and Training

(PRACTICE NAME) will ensure that employees and staff members with access to ePHI receive HIPAA Security Training and periodic security updates.[HIPAA 164.308(a)(5).]

I. Password Management

All covered components will adhere to the (PRACTICE NAME)'s Information Security Policy and Procedures regarding passwords on systems managing ePHI, as they are stronger than HIPAA requirements. In addition, passwords must be forced to change periodically, and must be changed immediately if compromised. [Addresses HIPAA Section 164.308(a)(5).]

J. Security Incident Procedures

The Compliance Officer will be (PRACTICE NAME)'s contact person for receiving information related to suspected or known incidents of unauthorized access to ePHI or loss of ePHI. The Compliance Officer will investigate and mitigate, to the extent practicable, any harmful effects of security incidents that are known, and will document any known security incidents and their outcomes. [HIPAA Section 164.308(a)(5).]

K. Contingency Plan

(PRACTICE NAME) will maintain a Contingency Plan for responding to system emergencies, which will include procedures for creating and maintaining backups of ePHI and restoring any data lost due to such an emergency. Each covered component will identify any critical business processes necessary and maintain its own procedures for enabling such processes to continue if essential.

L. Evaluation

The Compliance Officer will perform periodic evaluations, at least annually, to determine compliance with the HIPAA Security Rule and to ensure continued viability in light of environmental or operational changes that could affect the security of ePHI. [HIPAA Section 164.308(a)(8).]

M. Business Associate Contracts and Other Arrangements

(PRACTICE NAME) will enter into Business Associate Agreements with any third-party vendor ("Business Associate") it permits to create, receive, maintain, or transmit ePHI on the (PRACTICE NAME) behalf to ensure that the Business Associate will appropriately safeguard the information. Such contracts will provide that the Business Associate will (1) implement administrative, physical, and technical safeguards to reasonably protect the confidentiality, integrity, and availability of ePHI it has access to; (2) ensure that agents, including subcontractors, agree to implement reasonable and appropriate safeguards to protect ePHI; (3) report to the (PRACTICE NAME) any security incidents of which it becomes aware; and (4) terminate such contract upon request by the (PRACTICE NAME) and return or destroy all ePHI it maintains; and (5) comply with all requirements of business associates set forth in HIPAA Final Rule published on January 25, 2013.

IV. **Physical Safeguards**

A. Facility Access Controls

(PRACTICE NAME) will ensure that access to facilities housing ePHI are appropriately safeguarded against unauthorized physical access, tampering, or theft, while ensuring that properly authorized access is allowed. [HIPAA Section 164.310(a)(1).]

B. Workstation Use

(PRACTICE NAME)'s employee or staff member with authorized access to ePHI, will be assigned a specific workstation in which he/she is allowed to access such ePHI. These workstations will have appropriate security controls in place to prevent unauthorized access to ePHI. This extends to the use of laptop or home computers. [HIPAA Section 164.310 (b).]

C. Workstation Security

(PRACTICE NAME)'s employees or staff members with authorized access to ePHI will have their workstation locations set to eliminate or minimize the possibility of unauthorized access to ePHI. Workstations will be set with inactivity timeouts and use password-protected screen savers. [HIPAA Section 164.310 (c).]

D. Device and Media Controls

Laptop workstations will not be utilized for accessing ePHI without proper security and firewall protection, and only when permission has been granted by the Compliance Officer to access ePHI from such a workstation. ePHI should not be stored on any computer hard drive or other storage unit such as CDs or thumb drives without the approval of the Compliance Officer and appropriate steps taken to ensure data has been properly protected. Any medium used to store ePHI, such as for backup and recovery, if being disposed of, must be discarded or reused in a manner that prevents data recovery. [HIPAA Section 164.310 (d)(1).]

E. Mobile Device Policy

(PRACTICE NAME) utilizes a Mobile Device Policy that applies to all employees and staff members who bring personal electronic devices into (PRACTICE NAME)'s facilities.

V. Technical Safeguards

A. Access Control

Security controls will be established to ensure that access to systems containing ePHI will be allowed only to those employees who have been granted access rights. A unique user name will be used by each individual who is provided access to systems to enable identifying and tracking user identity. Emergency access procedures will be established to allow emergency access to systems necessary to continue business operations when needed. Workstations and applications will be programmed to automatically log out when inactivity has exceeded a set period of time established by each covered component, not to exceed 15 minutes. A mechanism for encrypting and decrypting data will be implemented when ePHI is transferred to/from systems not controlled by the (PRACTICE NAME). [HIPAA Section 164.312 (a)(1).]

B. Audit Controls

An audit process will be established to examine logged information to assist in identifying suspicious data-access activities. Audit logs will capture information on systems managing ePHI, including user access and activity, exception reports, dormant account reports, failed login reports, and unauthorized user access attempts. [HIPAA Section 164.312 (b).]

C. Integrity

Data will be protected from improper alteration or destruction through encryption and proper backup storage. [HIPAA Section 164.312 (c)(1).]

D. Person or Entity Authentication

Controls will be established to verify that a person seeking access to systems containing ePHI is the actual individual authorized. [HIPAA Section 164.312 (d).]

E. Transmission Security

Each covered component should have controls in place that ensure that the integrity of ePHI is maintained when in transit. Secure transmission mechanisms that encrypt ePHI as well as confirm that data integrity has been maintained should be used. The use of email for transmitting ePHI should be avoided; if required, emails with ePHI should be encrypted. [Addresses HIPAA Section 164.312(e)(1).]

F. Information Security

Individuals who access, receive, or otherwise handle or control ePHI on (PRACTICE NAME) systems will do so securely and responsibly. In addition to the directives specified in the HIPAA Security Rule, in (PRACTICE NAME) policies, and in department or area procedures, these individuals are expected to exercise good judgment in maintaining the security of all ePHI.

VI.   Civil and Criminal Penalties

Every employee and staff member of (PRACTICE NAME) with access to ePHI is required to adhere to all HIPAA mandates and any future additions or alterations to them. Under federal law, violations of the HIPAA privacy rule may result in civil monetary penalties of up to $50,000per violation and up to $1,500,000 for violations of the same issue in a calendar year. Criminal penalties may apply in some circumstances.

Appendix 5

PHOTOGRAPH AND VIDEO RELEASE

I, _____, (patient's name), hereby grant (PRACTICE NAME) and their successors and assigns, the right to use photographs, video clips, or other electronic images (collectively here after photographs) of me. I understand that I do not have any intellectual property rights in or to these images.

The usage of these photographs and/or digital images will be limited to:

    a. Medical purposes related to case.
    b. Scientific purposes, including seminars and medical articles.
    c. Before and after photo album (digital or printed) for cosmetic patients to view in the offices.
    d. Before and after photographs and/or digital images to be posted on websites such as YouTube or Facebook.
    e. Before and after photographs and/or digital images to be included on the practice's website for cosmetic surgery.

I understand I will not be identified explicitly by name in any use. That said, I also understand that in some circumstances the photographs may portray features that will make my identity recognizable. Hence, I understand while efforts will be made to balance my interest in privacy with the intended use, it is impossible to guarantee a third party will never be able to connect the photograph with my identity.

(PRACTICE NAME) need not approach me again for authorization to use these photographs unless the usage differs from that listed above. If I do not revoke this authorization, it will expire 10 years from the date written below.

If I ask (PRACTICE NAME) to terminate use of these photographs and/or digital images, I will do so in writing and communicated to (PRACTICE NAME) and recognize that it will likely take a reasonable time period to accomplish. For example, to remove such photographs from a web site, (PRACTICE NAME) will need to coordinate with a third-party webmaster.

Further, termination of prospective use of photographs and/or digital images may have no effect on prior distribution, such as the case with medical journals. A published journal, for example, cannot be "recalled."

I hold (PRACTICE NAME) harmless from any liability related to use of these photographs and/or digital images for the purposes outlined above. I further hold (PRACTICE NAME) harmless for any third-party use of these photographs unrelated to direct, immediate, and proximate action by (PRACTICE NAME).

This release and authorization does not conflict with any existing commitment on my part.

I understand that (PRACTICE NAME) is not obligated to make use of its rights set forth herein.

Copyright to photographs and/or digital images are retained by (PRACTICE NAME).

Patient Signature: _____   Date_____

Witness Signature:_____   Date_____

Appendix 6

SOCIAL MEDIA POLICY OF (PRACTICE NAME)

In recent years, social networking sites and blogs such as Facebook, YouTube, and Twitter have become part of our culture. Social networking sites and blogs can be a tremendous source of information and entertainment. Unfortunately, they can also be misused. What follows is (PRACTICE NAME)'s Social Media Policy. Employees of (PRACTICE NAME) should remember that the same basic policies apply in social media spaces as they do in other areas of their lives. The purpose of this policy is to help employees understand how (PRACTICE NAME)'s policies apply to these newer technologies for communication.

A. EXTENT OF POLICY

(PRACTICE NAME) believes that any communication referencing (PRACTICE NAME)'s employees and patients is information associated with (PRACTICE NAME). This policy does not apply to Internet activities that are not associated with (PRACTICE NAME) and are purely personal in nature.

B. TECHNOLOGY COVERED BY THIS POLICY

Because of the emerging nature of social media platforms and blogs, this policy does not attempt to name every current and emerging platform. Rather, the policy applies to those listed as examples below and to other platforms available and emerging, including social networking sites and sites with user-generated content. Examples of such platforms include: 1) Twitter, 2) Facebook, 3) MySpace, 4) YouTube, 5) Yelp.com, 6) RateMDs.com, 7) Angie's List, and 8) Instagram.

C. POLICY FOR ON-LINE PROFESSIONAL OR PERSONAL BEHAVIOR AND ACTIVITIES

1. You are prohibited from posting any content that is protected health information (PHI), including patient images, on any social media site or blog.
2. You are prohibited from using any social media site or blog to provide medical advice or medical commentary that in any way references (PRACTICE NAME) or your employment with (PRACTICE NAME).
3. You are prohibited from violating any local, state, federal, or international laws and regulations, including but not limited to copyright and intellectual property laws regarding any content that you transmit (by uploading posting, emailing, or otherwise) that is unlawful, disruptive, threatening, profane, abusive, harassing, embarrassing, impinges upon another person's privacy, racist, hateful, defamatory, libelous, or otherwise objectionable as solely determined by (PRACTICE NAME) and at (PRACTICE NAME)'s discretion.

4. You are prohibited from impersonating any person or entity or falsely stating or otherwise misrepresenting your affiliation with a person or entity.

5. You are prohibited from transmitting any material (by uploading, posting, emailing, or otherwise) that you do not have a right to make available under any law or contractual or fiduciary relationship.

6. You are prohibited from attempting to collect, collecting, and/or storing personal data about (PRACTICE NAME)'s employees or patients without their prior written consent.

7. You are prohibited from endorsing any product or service or taking any action that may be construed as political lobbying, campaigning, or solicitation, or take an stance on a position of any legislation or law in a manner that implicates, connotes, or references (PRACTICE NAME).

D. VIOLATION OF SOCIAL MEDIA POLICY

Violation of any portion of (PRACTICE NAME)'s Social Media Policy is inappropriate and may result in disciplinary action up to and including termination of employment. Any violation of this policy should immediately be reported to the (PRACTICE) Compliance Officer.

You agree that any claim dispute relating to your posting of any content on a social media platform or blog on the Internet shall be construed in accordance with the laws of the State of (PRACTICE STATE) without regard to its conflict of law provisions and that you agree to be bound and subject to the exclusive jurisdiction of local, state, or federal courts located in (PRACTICE STATE).

You shall defend, indemnify, and hold (PRACTICE NAME) and its respective officers/directors, employees, successors, and assigns, harmless from and against any and all losses, claims, damages, settlements, costs, and liabilities of any nature whatsoever (including reasonable attorney fees) as a result of or in any way connected with your posting of any content to a social media platform and/or blog.

E. POLICY AMENDMENTS

This Policy may be updated from time to time. To remain compliant, (PRACTICE NAME) suggests that you review its Social Media Policy at regular intervals. Any questions or concerns relating to this Social Media Policy or amendments to it should be directed to (PRACTICE NAME).

F. TERM OF POLICY

This Policy is effective immediately and survives termination of employment with (PRACTICE NAME).

SO AGREED AND UNDERSTOOD THIS _____ DAY OF _____, 20__.

_____ [EMPLOYEE]

Appendix 7

MOBILE DEVICE POLICY

I.   Definitions

For purposes of this policy, a mobile device includes any electronic device that captures, stores, or transmits data. Examples of mobile devices include cell phones, smart phones, tablets, and other such devices.

II.   Applicability of This Policy

(PRACTICE NAME), hereafter referred to as "employer," makes every effort to protect the health information of its patients and comply with both state and federal privacy regulations. Mobile devices offer tremendous benefits for users and have become a reality of daily life. However, these devices also pose the potential for security violations, unattended data breaches, or data loss. This policy is designed to provide guidance to employees of (PRACTICE NAME) on appropriate uses of private mobile devices.

This policy applies to any mobile device brought by an employee to (PRACTICE NAME)'s premises. It also applies to any employee's use of such device to access information of employer or to in any way perform duties associated with their employment at (PRACTICE NAME).

III.   Security Requirements

All employees of (PRACTICE NAME) who use a mobile device in a way described above are responsible for securing their device to prevent sensitive data from being lost, inappropriately accessed, corrupted, or otherwise compromised. If an employee believes that his or her mobile device has been stolen, lost, hacked, or otherwise compromised, this belief should be immediately reported to the (PRACTICE NAME) Compliance Officer.

In order to protect the mobile device, employees are to:

    a. Have a password or personal identification number PIN consisting of at least four characters. Security experts recommend a combination of both letters and numerals.

    b. Configure the mobile device so the password/PIN must be entered to activate the functionality of the device after 15 minutes of inactivity or less.

    c. Load apps or software, if possible, to remotely locate the device should it be misplaced.

    d. Load apps or software, if possible, to remotely "wipe" or delete information from the device should it be misplaced.

    e. Enable encryption on the device if possible.

    f. Keep the device charged; the loss of power can potentially cause stored data to be erased.

    g. Regularly back up the device and keep it up to date with the latest iteration and the latest software and application iteration and updates.

    h. Install anti-virus software if possible.

IX. Prohibited Uses

    a. Camera. Many mobile devices now include cameras. This is a particular concern in the healthcare arena. Employees are never to take photographs of patients with their mobile device. Further, employees are never to use mobile devices to take photographs of patients' medical records, charts, test results, x-rays, scans, or other studies of a patient. It is prohibited to take a photograph of any portion or part of a patient's body with an employee's mobile device with or without patient's approval. Any photographs of a patient that need to be taken for medical purposes shall be taken by a camera supplied by an employer to an employee and shall be recorded in that patient's medical record. The use of an employee's personal device for photographing a patient or any portion of a patient with or without patient's approval is grounds for immediate dismissal.

    b. Texting. Employees texting information to or about any patient of (PRACTICE NAME) is prohibited unless the text is done via approved, encrypted software pursuant to the HITECH Act. All electronic communications regarding patients must be encrypted, including includes texts. Should employees feel that it is necessary to the performance of their employment duties, employees should confirm with employer's Compliance Officer that the text software is appropriate and secure.

    c. Storage of patient data. Generally, patient data is not to be kept in any fashion on an employee's mobile device to the extent that it is accessed and temporarily stored on the employee's device. The patient's data is to be deleted at the first opportunity. Information captured on an employee's device that is of medical relevancy to a patient shall be transferred or transcribed into that patient's medical record. It is inappropriate and impermissible to house patient data for any length of time on an employee's personal device.

IV. Prohibited Locations for Use of Mobile Devices

Mobile devices can be a distraction. At no time are employee devices permitted in a room where a patient is undergoing an invasive procedure. Additionally, for technology reasons, employee devices are not permitted in the following locations _____.
Finally, employer deserves the right to prohibit or restrict employees from using a mobile device from time to time in different locations based upon patient safety and professionalism.

V. Alteration of the Above Policy

Employer reserves the right from time to time to alter, amend, delete, or supplement this Mobile Device Policy. If employee has a question as to his or her obligations under this policy or a subsequent iteration, that employee may consult (PRACTICE NAME)'s Compliance Officer. The above policy became effective on _____ day of _____, 20_____.

Appendix 8

DATA AND ELECTRONIC EQUIPMENT SANITATION AND DISPOSAL POLICY FOR (PRACTICE NAME)

Data equipment and sanitation disposal is the deliberate and permanent removal or destruction of the data printed or stored on a storage media device such as a hard drive. When the storage media device becomes obsolete or sensitive data is no longer needed, all sensitive data must effectively be destroyed either by shredding of paper or removal of the storage media before the device is reused or discarded. Sensitive data includes all protected health information (PHI) as the same is defined by federal law. This policy defines the appropriate destruction of sensitive data to be used by (PRACTICE NAME).

Reason for Policy

This policy ensures that sensitive data is not inappropriately released. (PRACTICE NAME) makes every effort to protect its patients' information and comply with all laws. Examples of laws related to this policy include, but are not limited to, the Health Insurance Portability and Accountability Act (HIPAA) and the Gramm Leach Bliley Act (GLBA). The policy protects sensitive data that could be kept on paper or stored in devices, including but not exclusive to desktop and laptop computer hard drives, removable storage devices (e.g., a CD, DVD, external hard drive, USB disk or flash drive), or any devices with storage capacity.

Responsible Officer of (PRATICE NAME)

The Compliance Officer for (PRACTICE NAME) is responsible for the maintenance of this policy and for responding to questions regarding this policy.

Who Is Governed by This Policy?

This policy applies to all individuals who have access to, use of, or control of sensitive data and PHI of (PRACTICE NAME). Those individuals covered include, but are not limited to, employees, contractors, consultants, and others working at (PRACTICE NAME).

Policy Text

This policy covers all information regardless of storage medium (e.g., paper, fiche, electronic tape, cartridge, disk, CD, DVD, external drive) and regardless of form (e.g., text, graphic video, voice). When sensitive documents and data are no longer required, they must be sanitized in accordance to the sanitation method below.

The data sanitization process involves the following steps:

- Assessing the sensitivity and security category of the stored data;
- Selecting the appropriate data sanitization method based on the category;
- Sanitizing the media; and
- Verifying the result.

See the Data Classification Policy for details of the three data classification categories:

- Category HS—Highest Sensitivity (Confidential/Sensitive Data)
- Category MS—Moderate Sensitivity (Internal/Official Use Only Data)
- Category NS—Not Sensitive (Public Data)

Based on this data classification, electronic data on magnetic storage and media devices should be sanitized using the following methods:

Categories HS and MS Sanitization Method

Use specialized data removal software to remove the data more robustly than simply deleting and/or reformatting the media device before the media device is reused. Examples of such data software removal software include Darik's Boot and Nuke and Blancco.

Note: If a computer was used to access sensitive information, there is a high likelihood that the system retained that information on the hard drive even after the user has exited the program. Therefore, always use the categories HS and MS sanitization method to cleanse the equipment prior to reuse and/or disposal.

Category NS Sanitization Method

The media should be reformatted before it is reused.

Multiple Categories Sanitation Method

When a storage media device contains data of multiple categories, use the sanitization method for categories HS and MS.

Disposal Process for Paper

Any paper document that contains sensitive data or PHI must be disposed of by shredding, burning, or chemically altering the document to the degree that it is no longer legible.

Disposal Process for Electronic Equipment

When discarding any equipment with a storage media device, always verify whether the device contains any data classified as Category HS or MS and then apply the appropriate data sanitization method. Remove the storage media device from the equipment, if possible, and discard it separately and more securely (e.g., disintegration and/or pulverization), making the device unsalvageable and unusable.

For discarding non-reusable media (e.g., CD+/-R, DVD+/-R, paper, fiche, etc.) that contains sensitive data, take steps to adequately destroy the media (e.g., disintegration, pulverization, or cross-cut shredding) to make the device physically unsalvageable and unusable.

Responsibilities

All individuals covered by this policy have a responsibility to protect the confidentiality, integrity, and availability of data stored or used by (PRACTICE NAME), irrespective of the media on which the data resides and regardless of format (e.g., in electronic, paper, or other physical form).

Failure to abide by this policy may lead to disciplinary action and/or sanctions up to and including discharge or dismissal in accordance to policy and procedures. Additionally, intentional negligence that results in breach of confidentiality of data that is protected by law, acts, or regulations can also result in criminal prosecution.

Adoption

The above policy was adopted this _____day of _____, 20__.

_____

(NAME), Compliance Officer